LIFE BEHIND THE MASK

LIFE BEHIND THE MASK
A SURGEON'S MEMOIR

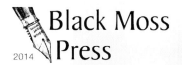
Black Moss Press
2014

DR. MICHAEL AKPATA

Copyright © Michael Akpata 2014

Akpata, Michael, author
    Life behind the mask : a surgeon's memoir / Dr. Michael Akpata.

ISBN 978-0-88753-542-0 (pbk.)

1. Akpata, Michael. 2. Surgeons--Canada--Biography. I. Title.

RD27.35.A46A3 2014   617.092   C2014-903999-9

Editing: Bob Meyer
Design & Layout: Jason Rankin

Published by Black Moss Press at 2450 Byng Road, Windsor, Ontario, N8W 3E8. Canada. Black Moss books are distributed in Canada and the U.S. by Fitzhenry & Whiteside. All orders should be directed there.

Fitzhenry & Whiteside
195 Allstate Parkway
Markham, ON
L3R 4T8

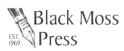

Black Moss would like to acknowledge the generous financial support from both the Canada Council for the Arts and the Ontario Arts Council.

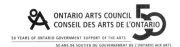
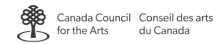
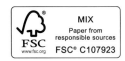

DEDICATION

I dedicate this book to the following people who have contributed to both my private and professional life.

DR. MURRAY GIROTTI

Dr. Girotti was both a good friend and my mentor. Unfortunately, he died at the early age of 62 at home on Sunday, December 26, 2010. He played a major role in my active interest in laparoscopic surgery which became a main part of my career. As a result of his tutorship, I undertook many advanced laparoscopic surgery courses. I was very sad to hear of his demise and my prayers go with his family.

DAVID THOMPSON - PRIME MINISTER OF BARBADOS

David Thompson was born on December 25, 1961 and died following an illness on October 23, 2010 at the early age of 48. He was a kind, gentle and compassionate man and undoubtedly one of my most reliable and trusted friends. My friendship with him was instrumental in my developing a special affection for the beautiful island of Barbados. He was the Prime Minister of Barbados during the last two years of his life and unfortunately died while still in office.

I first met him when he was the Minister of Finance for Barbados in 1994. Prior to that, his first cabinet appointment was that of the Minister of Community Development and Culture, a position which befitted his personality. It was a stroke of luck that I was introduced to him by Dr. Jerry Emtage and we quickly became friends.

There is a lot I could say about Mr. Thompson as a friend and a reliable politician, but this will require another book. We were so close that he asked me to be the godfather to his youngest daughter and I humbly accepted the offer. I sincerely miss him and my prayers go with his dear wife, Mara and his three children, including my goddaughter, Osa Marie.

MY FATHER

My father was dedicated to the education of his children and he made it his duty to teach us how to pray and become good Christians. I am forever grateful and indebted to him for the role he played in my life. May his soul rest in peace.

MY CHILDREN

My three children, Michael, Michelle and John, who saw very little of me when they were growing up because of my extreme commitment to my work, are the love of my life. I am very proud of their accomplishments in life and thank them for giving me four beautiful grandchildren, Reece, Regan, Ayla and Evan, whom I love dearly.

TABLE OF CONTENTS

Preface • 9
Chapter One • 11
Three-Piece Suit Affair
Chapter Two • 13
Why I Chose to Study Medicine
Chapter Three • 14
Why I Chose Canada
Chapter Four • 15
Secondary School Education
Chapter Five • 20
First Year at the University of Alberta
Chapter Six • 23
Admission into Medical School
Chapter Seven • 25
Second and Third Year of Medical School
Chapter Eight • 27
End of Fourth Year Medicine
Chapter Nine • 31
Rotating Internship
Chapter Ten • 32
First Year Residency Program
Chapter Eleven • 33
Second Year Residency Program
Chapter Twelve • 35
Associate Resident Year
Chapter Thirteen • 37
Fourth Year Residency
Chapter Fourteen • 39
Appointment as a Teaching Fellow
Chapter Fifteen • 40
Application to Grace Hospital Toronto
Chapter Sixteen • 41
Move to Windsor
Chapter Seventeen • 43
Beginning My Practice

Chapter Eighteen • 47
Hôtel Dieu 100 Year Anniversary
Chapter Nineteen • 51
Beginning of New Procedures
Chapter Twenty • 53
Age of Laparoscopy
Chapter Twenty One • 61
Training in Advanced Laparoscopy
Chapter Twenty Two • 64
Symposium on Minimal Access Surgery

PHOTO Gallery • 65

Chapter Twenty Three • 73
Society for Laparoscopic and Endoscopic Surgery
Chapter Twenty Four • 75
Post Graduate Course - Advanced Laparoscopy
Chapter Twenty Five • 79
CBC Television Interviews
Chapter Twenty Six • 80
Caribbean Connection
Chapter Twenty Seven • 87
Other Pioneering Innovators
Chapter Twenty Eight • 90
Hospital Committees
Chapter Twenty Nine • 91
Secretary to the Department of Surgery
Chapter Thirty • 94
Changes in Department of Surgery - Hôtel Dieu
Chapter Thirty One • 95
Sentinel Lymph Node Biopsy
Chapter Thirty Two • 96
Amalgamation of the Windsor Hospitals

Chapter Thirty Three • 98
McMaster University Health Sciences
Chapter Thirty Four • 101
Endoscopic Practice
Chapter Thirty Five • 104
Plans for Private Endoscopy Clinic
Chapter Thirty Six • 106
An unexpected event
Chapter Thirty Seven • 108
Good Samaritans in my Life
Chapter Thirty Eight • 110
History of the Benin Kingdom
Chapter Thirty Nine • 113
Family Background
Chapter Forty • 115
Family Upbringing
Chapter Forty One • 120
Primary School Education
Chapter Forty Two • 122
Relationship with Patients and Staff
Chapter Forty Three • 123
Reminiscing Over my Practice
Chapter Forty Four • 127
Passions in Life

Conclusion • 133

Acknowledgements • 135
Praise for Life Behind the Mask • 136

PREFACE

I have not written this book with a sense of pride but rather with trembling humility. It is a testament of what God gave me at birth and has nurtured throughout my life. My aim in writing this book is to bring forth my contributions to the changes that have taken place since my arrival in Windsor in the fields of General Surgery and Gastrointestinal Endoscopy.

It is also an attempt in all sincerity, to show what a person can do if one dedicates himself to his or her calling. The rest of the book reflects my early childhood and family life in Nigeria. I hope you will enjoy reading it. Much of my working life was spent with a surgeon's mask on my face. Though often my job entailed not being heard or seen, my actions, I hope, have spoken much louder than any words I could have uttered.

Also this book is a collection of successful and time tested recipes of my professional life. It will show that, 'learning is an active process and that we learn by doing', as George Bernard Shaw once said. It is also an attempt to emphasize the saying that the first half of one's life is used to build one's legitimacy. By all accounts, I feel I have fulfilled that objective, despite some difficult moments. The next step is for me to leave behind my legacy in the form of this book.

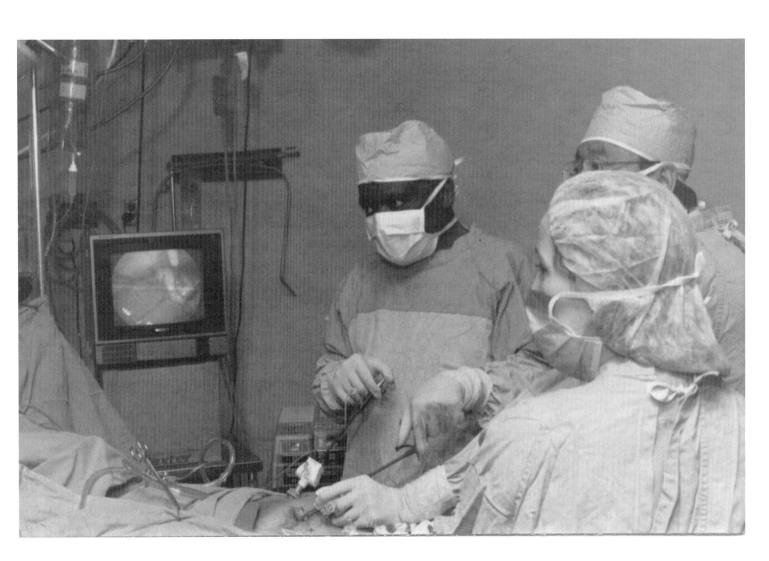

CHAPTER ONE
THREE-PIECE SUIT AFFAIR

It was in the autumn of 1960 that I arrived in Canada. To be precise, it was a day in September when I bade farewell to my family and friends in Nigeria, my native country in West Africa, and headed for the University of Alberta in Edmonton, Alberta, Canada. I boarded the British Overseas Airways Corporation plane, now called British Airways, in Lagos, Nigeria, for my long flight. I was anxious as this was the first time I would be leaving my home country and full of anticipation as I was determined to attain a university education in medicine abroad.

I was only 18 years old at the time. My father ensured that I travel in a three-piece suit because, as a university student, I was to be a model for both my family and my country. In those days, this was common attire and a hallmark of a university student in Nigeria.

My country was a vast colony of the British Empire with a population of 60 million but has since grown to 175 million. Nigerians are highly motivated, intelligent and hard working people who cherish education. When I left Nigeria, the country had a bright future, especially following the discovery of oil in great quantities. It would soon gain independence from Britain.

Nigeria only had one university for the entire country called the University College of Ibadan, patterned on the heels of London University, England and therefore, it was a privilege and an honor to be admitted for training there. The students were expected to be well groomed when on or off campus grounds. But, my interest was to attend a university abroad, either in England or preferably in North America.

After the country attained independence from the British, in October 1960, the new government decided to set up a number of universities, technical colleges and high-quality medical schools. These plans were still in the preliminary stages when I left the country in September of that year.

When I arrived at the University of Alberta campus on that first evening, I soon realized I was completely out of place in my three-piece suit. Here I was in the midst of students wearing jeans, cowboy boots and cowboy hats, laughing, joking, drinking and generally having a great time at the tuck shop. When I saw the students in their attire, no one was dressed as I had expected and this was very strange.

My mind was in a state of confusion. I asked myself, "Michael, what have you done, where are you and what are you doing here with these people? Why did you leave home expecting university students to be like those you left behind in Nigeria, a poor and underdeveloped country? After all, this is Canada, advanced and rich in resources."

The strange stares I received from the students gathered around the tuck shop made me feel uncomfortable and completely out of place. The voice within me said, "Go back home, you do not belong here. This is not what you expected."

Coming from the so-called 'jungle of Africa' in a three-piece suit to attend a prominent Canadian university, I felt as though many of the students were making fun of me. I felt odd. I came from a country where I had never experienced prejudice or racism.

It made more sense to me when I was told that this was the 'frosh weekend' when the new students were able to wear their local attire and have fun with each other before the university classes began.

In retrospect, I can understand the cool welcome that I received, since the 1960's were still a very turbulent time especially in the United States between black and white races.

Many articles appeared in papers about the social upheaval, riots and violence against one another. Even university students were involved and some were killed. I was one of the few black students who attended the University of Alberta at that time.

Later, I learned that I was the first African student to attend this medical school from the beginning of the course throughout including internship and residency in general surgery. Following my postgraduate training, I was appointed to the position of a Teaching Fellow for one year. It was indeed a great honor for me.

CHAPTER TWO
WHY I CHOSE TO STUDY MEDICINE

There was an interesting situation which occurred to me when I was five or six years old that had a great impact on me to study medicine when I grew up. My father had several friends, some Nigerian and others British, because of his many business associations.

On one occasion, I took ill and my father sent me with his driver to the hospital to see one of his very close friends who was an Internist from Ireland. He had given me a written note to present to the doctor asking him to examine me.

To understand the events that followed my arrival at the hospital, it is important for me to explain why I was sent directly to him instead of being sent to the emergency department as usual.

Although the hospital in the city where we lived in Benin had a good emergency department, it was always filled. Patients would sit on benches in order of arrival and continue to slide towards the nurse attendant who would then decide if they needed to be seen by a regular physician or a specialist.

This used to take hours before the patient would be seen by a qualified doctor and my father did not want me to stay in the emergency department for so long. I was taken directly to his friend's waiting area by my father's driver.

Whenever I went to the hospital in the past with my father, we were seated in his special waiting room and were attended to quickly. However, on this occasion the room was filled with many prominent people. After about half an hour the dispenser, a senior male nurse, decided that there were too many people in the waiting room and it was time for him to remove the non privileged.

He started to ask the status of each patient in the room. As it turned out, everyone he questioned was allowed to stay because of who they were. For example, when he asked the lady sitting next to me, she said that she was the wife of the Superintendant of Schools and with that she was allowed to sit down. When he came to me, a five or six year old boy, I said to him, "I am my father's son, a friend of the Irish Internist."

At this point, he told me and my father's driver to get out of the room in spite of the fact that he had seen me there before on several occasions with my dad. He kept yelling, "Out, out, out."

We quickly left the waiting lounge and headed home to tell my father what had happened. On my way home, I made a life-altering decision. When I grew up, I would become a doctor and never turn anybody away from my practice based on their income or status.

When I got home and relayed my experiences to my dad, he immediately jumped into the car and took me back to the clinic because he saw the urgency. We went back into the very same waiting room and ran into the male nurse who had thrown me out.

When he saw my dad, he was all smiles and asked him how he could help. At the same time my dad's friend, the Internist, came out of his room and took us into his office right away. The incident stuck with me throughout my study of medicine and the 32 years working as a surgeon in Windsor, Ontario. This lesson taught me that all patients would require my undivided attention regardless of their appearance or social status.

CHAPTER THREE
WHY I CHOSE CANADA

In 1959, someone asked me why I wanted to attend a Canadian university instead of going to Britain like most of the other Nigerian students. I told him that I had made up my mind a long time ago. During my high school training at King's College, we were taught the history and geography of Canada, the United States and especially Great Britain since Nigeria was still a colony of the British.

Most Nigerians knew nothing about Canada just as I'm sure that Canadians knew nothing about Nigeria. However, we had been taught that Canada was a vast and unique country with great potential.

Secondly, it was a new frontier for Nigerians and to some extent other Africans who wanted to go overseas to study without the trappings of colonialism. Most of my classmates and relatives went to Britain to take postgraduate or university training but I was not interested in going there.

A province in Canada with unusual names like Crow's Nest Pass, Kicking Horse Pass and Medicine Hat aroused my spirit of adventure.

During one of our class parties, my science teacher who was from Bristol, England asked me why I had chosen Canada and especially Alberta, instead of the renowned medical school in Bristol to study medicine.

I didn't know that during his last visit on holidays in England he had actually helped to secure admission opportunities for three students in my class at King's College, to study medicine in Bristol.

To my surprise I was one of them.

The other two students were very happy, but I was not interested and so I kept quiet. Obviously he was disappointed, since Bristol University was his alma mater and very reputable in England.

Then he said, "Tell me, Akpata, why would you refuse such a wonderful opportunity and instead choose to go to the University of Alberta? What do you know about Canada that intrigues you so much?"

That is when I recited those three strange place names. One of the staff members present during this discussion heard what we were talking about. While looking straight at me, he said, "I have never heard of that place. Maybe it was discovered by the late Prince Albert." He continued to stare at me and with his typical English accent, he said, "Pity", while shaking his head and walking away.

I had done research into Canadian universities and my first choice was McGill which was renowned for neuro-science and neuro-surgery. This was very well known in Nigeria. I wrote a letter of application to all the universities in the capitals of all the provinces in Canada, including McGill University.

I was not aware that Laval University was the one located in the capital of Quebec rather than McGill which is located in Montréal. Unfortunately, I had addressed my request for application to McGill University in Quebec City instead of Montreal.

I finally received a response from Laval University admitting me into their program as long as I could speak French. But I knew that my French was not good enough and so I decided not to respond to the letter. I kept waiting for a response from McGill but none was forthcoming.

The next letter I received was from the University of Alberta confirming my admission. Included in the letter was the name of the person who was going to wait for me at the airport, my course content and also my room number at the Athabasca Hall residence. I was honored to receive all of these materials from this university.

On that day, I decided that this would be the best choice for me even though I was still disappointed that I did not get a response from McGill.

My father was pleased to see me get admitted into a university abroad and was not upset that I had chosen to go to Canada instead of Bristol, in spite of the fact that most of my brothers, sisters and cousins had trained in England. Although I was only 18, he was willing to allow me to go to a place so far away that I had never visited before. He said that I would get to know another part of the world which would be helpful to me.

He assumed that all of us would be returning home after our training and had even offered to build us a hospital named Akpata Memorial Hospital, where we could work.

CHAPTER FOUR
SECONDARY SCHOOL EDUCATION

King's College was founded in 1909 by the British when Nigeria was still their colony. It was called the Eton's College of Africa as it was patterned after Eton's College in London, England and was designed by the British with the aim of training future

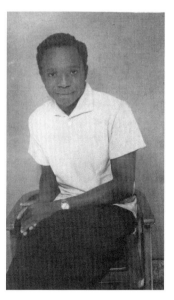

Michael Akpata, age 11, first year at King's College, Lagos.

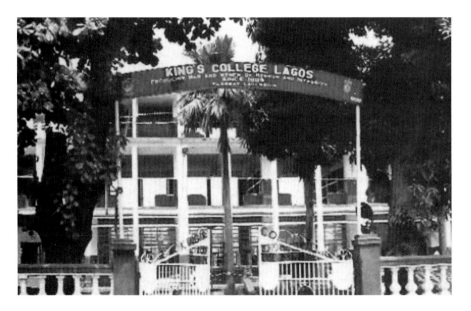

King's College, Lagos. Founded in 1909.

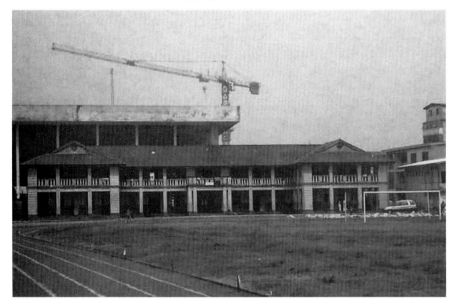

Hyde-Johnson's house, Michael's residence at King's College.

leaders of Nigeria. It was a unique boarding school with strict moral, ethical and intellectual codes.

Fortunately, it was a publicly funded boarding school with English traditions. With the exception of three teachers, the majority were recruited from British universities by the government. The teachers were called 'Masters'. The final graduating examinations were called the Cambridge Higher School Certificate Examinations as they were the same ones written by the British students on the same level each year.

Admission to King's College was by an entrance examination held each year across the country. Each province was assigned a specific number of students to be admitted based on their performance in the common entrance examination. Only the students with aptitude for higher education and possibly future leadership were accepted into the college.

My father attended King's College from 1915 to 1919. I was one of those fortunate enough to have been admitted at the age of eleven. At last count, at least 20 members of the Akpata family have been trained in this institution up to Grade 13, called the 'upper class'. It became an Akpata tradition to attend King's College. There was no other institution which had the same stature and ideals of this college. Other members of the family attended first-class boarding schools elsewhere in the country.

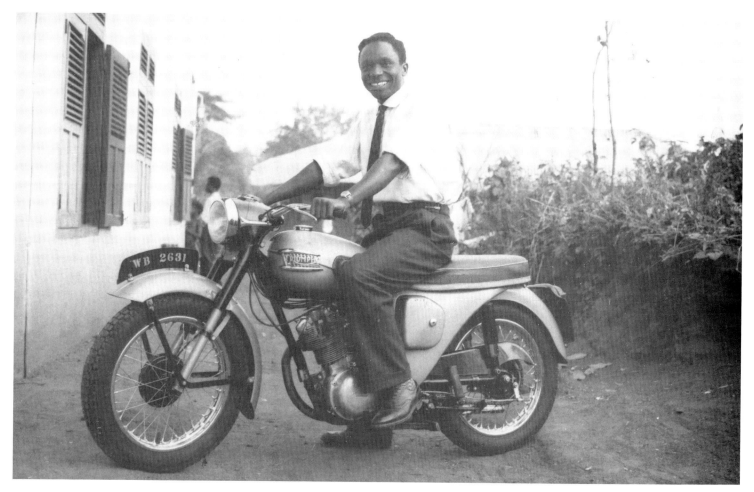

Michael on a motorcycle in front of the family home.

When I was at King's College, two other members of my family (my cousins) were also attending. We were identified numerically as Akpata 1, Akpata 2, and Akpata 3. Number one was Solomon or Sunny for short, I was number two and Henry was number three. Sunny was two years ahead of me and I was three years ahead of Henry. When Sunny left, I became number one and Henry became number two. But when I left, Henry did not have any junior member of the family attending making him the only Akpata.

There were four boarding houses at King's College; Harman's, Panes', McKee-Wright's and Hyde-Johnson's. Each house had an equitable number of students residing in it and each house had a specific color of T-shirt for casual wear and for athletic competitions. A school teacher called

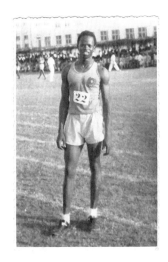

Sunny, Michael's cousin, at the 1957 Interhouse Sports, King's College.

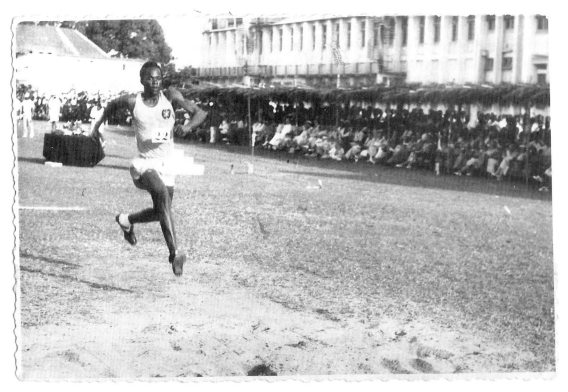

Sunny in 1957 doing triple jump, King's College, Lagos.

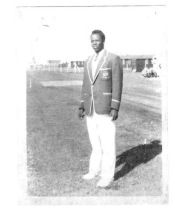

Sunny at the British Empire and Commonwealth Games, Cardiff, Wales 1958.

the 'House Master' was assigned to each house. I was a resident of Hyde-Johnson's house as were all my family members who had attended King's College. This was part of the college tradition. Our house color was red and the other house colors were respectively, green, blue and yellow.

Loyalty to one's house was an absolute must and created healthy competition among the students.

There were eight school prefects who were appointed by the principal and teachers and one of them was chosen as the school captain. The role of the school prefect was to ensure that all students obeyed the school's bylaws while the school captain was the 'commander-in chief'. Any complaints from school prefects were reported to him and it was his role to deal with the problem. Otherwise he would pass it on to the principal. Members of each house elected their own house captain. His responsibility was to ensure that members of his house carried out their daily duties.

I was appointed as a school prefect, and also was elected as house captain of Hyde-Johnson's house during my last year. This arrangement was the first step in learning democratic process which was the cornerstone of King's College discipline.

There was a lot of competition between the houses regarding cleanliness, attention to bell calls and generally following college rules. Each morning at 7 am, the bell would ring for everyone to be up and out of his bed in preparation for having a shower and breakfast. There was always a first and second bell and by 7:45 am every student had to have had a shower, have his bed made and be standing beside the bed in his dormitory for inspection.

This inspection was carried out by a school prefect from another house on a rotational basis. Following this examination, appropriate marks were awarded to each house based on the level of cleanliness of the students, their punctuality at their bedside and each student's level of care of his bed.

The best house got three points, the next best received two points and the third got one point. The house with the worst performance had no points. At the end of the week, the points were then totaled and an announcement was made in the dining hall of the positions held by each house during the week. Points were also deducted from each house whose members arrived at the dining hall late and the total was given to each house captain every week.

Following this, the house captain of each individual house would go through the point system and each house had a way of punishing the worst offenders by making them do more house cleaning jobs. Any recurrent offender would then be subject to punishment by his house captain. Usually this involved making the culprit write an essay on any particular topic chosen by the house captain. For example, this could involve 'the role of punctuality in one's daily routine'.

Another very important aspect was the inter-house sports competitions which included track and field, soccer, field hockey, cricket, pole vaulting, and relay races. Each year, there was an inter-house track and field competition to which family members and dignitaries were invited to watch. I participated in the 100 meter run, pole vaulting, hurdles and high jump. There was a gold cup awarded to the house that won the highest number of points.

The Akpata family was known for participating in all of these sporting events at some point during their training in the college.

My cousin, Sunny, was an exceptional athlete and was so accomplished that he actually represented Nigeria in the 1958 Commonwealth Games in Cardiff, Wales. During his university years he represented Nigeria in the 1960 Olympic Games in

CHAPTER FIVE
FIRST YEAR AT THE UNIVERSITY OF ALBERTA

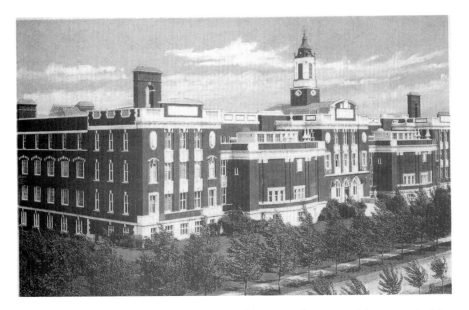

Postcard image of The University of Alberta Medical Building.

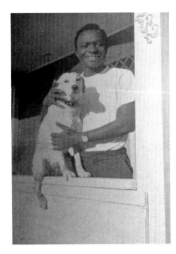

Michael at home in Alberta.

Upon my arrival in Edmonton, I was assigned to Athabaska Hall as my residence. There were several residences on campus each with a leader similar to the house captain at King's College. The president of Athabaska Hall was Jim Coutts, a law student, who later became secretary to Lester B. Pearson and eventually principal secretary to Pierre Elliott Trudeau.

Nigeria gained independence from Britain in 1960. There was a restriction imposed on people of my age from leaving and going abroad to study medicine because there was a plan afoot to build several medical schools in the near future. My main interest was in medicine but due to this restriction, the only way for me to leave the country with a scholarship was to apply for dentistry since there were no dental schools in the country at that time.

I had no choice but to register in the pre-dental first year class which was a similar requirement to the pre-medical class.

This first year went very well for me. In fact it was so good that in one of our examinations, I topped the physics class and also made the Dean's Honor list. I qualified to be admitted into the Department of Dentistry in September of 1961. The first year of dentistry was merely an introduction into the

Rome and later in the 1964 Olympics in Tokyo, Japan. His specialty was long jump and triple jump.

We were all very proud of him as an athlete and as a member of our family. Although the rest of us did not attend Commonwealth or Olympic Games, we were representatives of our college at numerous athletic events against other secondary schools in Nigeria and Ghana. Sunny and I, as well as other members of the Akpata family were awarded colors for our winning performances in cricket.

program including tooth carving and taking impressions of teeth under the supervision of a dental technologist.

Overall I found dentistry not very satisfying and actually quite boring. It did not take me long to realize that medicine would be a greater challenge and was definitely what I wanted to do. Since I already had the scholarship from the Nigerian government for dentistry, the question facing me then was how to pay for school fees if I transferred out of dentistry and into medicine.

I approached the Dean of Medicine to request admission into the Faculty of Medicine the following year starting in September 1962. He warned me I could not switch from a major faculty like Dentistry without the consent of the Dean of Dentistry.

After a long discussion, he agreed to give me an application form for entry into medicine but he insisted that I should speak to the Dean of Dentistry of my intention to change faculties.

I did this and although the Dean of Dentistry was not happy, he told me it was my life.

I knew it would be very difficult for me to compete with all the students who had already taken the second year pre-medical training and also with other applicants who had their first or second degrees and were waiting to be admitted into the Faculty of Medicine.

I wrote to the Nigerian High Commission in New York telling them of my plan to change into medicine and that I would like to keep my Nigerian scholarship. In less than one week came the response that this was not acceptable and my scholarship was withdrawn.

I went on summer holidays from June to September of 1962 while waiting to find out if I would be allowed to transfer into medicine. I decided to spend time with my cousin Sunny who was a student at Michigan

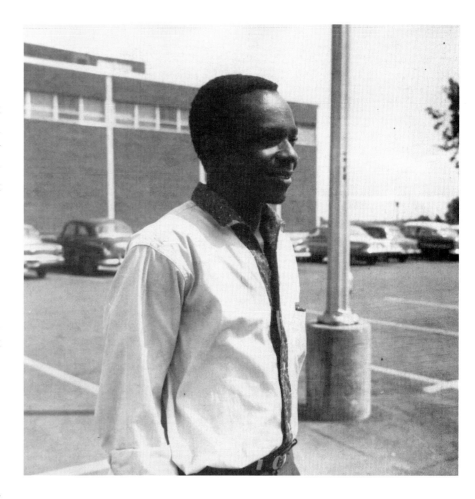

Michael in first year, University of Alberta.

State University in East Lansing, Michigan. He was happy to see me and helped me get odd jobs during my stay to earn some money before my return to Edmonton. Among the projects I got involved in was picking weeds at the university agricultural farm. But because of the effects of bending down for hours, I decided not to continue with this job.

One of the professors of linguistic studies at the university offered me a job to help him translate a book to a local Nigerian dialect called Bini. This is a language spoken in Benin City and the surrounding province of the same name.

I was no longer versed in this language. I had been away from Nigeria too long and more importantly, when I was in my secondary school at King's College, we were forbidden to speak in our local dialect and were restricted to speaking only English.

This was to prevent friction among the students from different ethnic backgrounds. The explanation given for this was that King's College was designed to train all students to be future leaders of the country and there would be no tolerance for tribalism. I was not able to give the professor the help he needed.

Instead, I decided to start mowing lawns in the area around the university campus. I made a deal with my cousin's landlady to rent her lawnmower for a fixed amount daily and then went from door to door to the houses on campus offering to mow lawns on a weekly basis for five dollars per hour or a flat fee of twenty dollars. This was quite an opportunity for me to make some money before I went back to the University of Alberta. I enjoyed doing it daily from 9 am to 4 pm and saw it as good exercise.

One day while mowing the lawn of one of my customers, his wife asked me if I would be willing to climb up to the roof and clean the debris out of the eave troughs. During the process, I lost my balance and fell but luckily sustained no injuries.

The lady quickly came out of her house and asked if I was all right. She then proceeded to ask me if I had any insurance protection for my yard mowing and cleaning which I did not. At that point, she told me to stop working, paid me in full and told me not to come back again to her house.

Following this episode, I decided to stop the lawn mowing business and return to Edmonton to spend the rest of the holidays resting and preparing for my medical training if I was accepted. I bought my cousin's car for a nominal fee and drove back through Michigan and the rest of the country toward Edmonton.

While driving through the small towns in Saskatchewan, I was listening to music and preoccupied with what I would face when I arrived back at the university campus in terms of my next course. Suddenly, a police car stopped me.

The officer immediately took me to a store nearby owned by a man who happened to be a Notary Public and I was charged with speeding. As I was not a resident of that province, they decided that a quasi-court session should be held immediately. I apologized and admitted that I probably was driving too fast but that was not good enough.

I was fined one hundred and fifty dollars to be paid immediately or else I would 'sleep in Hollywood' from then on until I paid the fine. I was shocked by the extreme manner in which this case was handled, but luckily, I had enough money with me to pay the fine. I was relieved to get out and proceeded to drive on to Edmonton at a much reduced speed. Lesson learned.

CHAPTER SIX
ADMISSION INTO MEDICAL SCHOOL

I was happily surprised to find that I had been admitted into the Faculty of Medicine at the University of Alberta. I had earned some money from my jobs during the holidays but it was not enough to live on and pay my tuition fees. I only had enough to pay fees for the first term and not enough to cover my books and residential fees.

My only option was to approach the administration of the university to tell them about my plight and ask if there was a grant for which I could apply. Within a few days of this discussion, I received a call to meet with the secretary. When we met he told

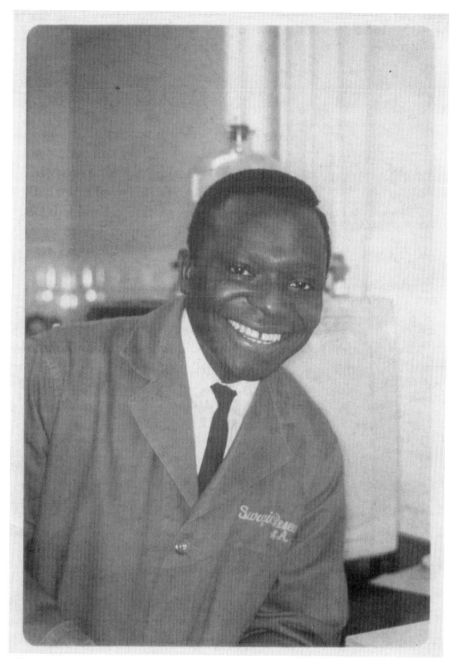

Michael Akpata spent time in the University of Alberta's surgical medical research lab (SMRI).

me that, based on my performance in the previous two years of study at the university, the administration had decided to grant me a special scholarship on a yearly basis. It was the first time this scholarship had been given to anybody and was called the University of Alberta Campus Special Award.

The terms and conditions of this special scholarship were as follows:

- The scholarship was to be awarded yearly, based on my performance scholastically. It would be extended each year as long as I maintained a good academic standing for the four years it would take to complete my entire medical training.
- The scholarship would pay for my books and tuition in addition to a living allowance of $250 per month.
- The scholarship would be withdrawn if I did not maintain my academic standing.

I cannot describe how ecstatic I felt to be the first student awarded this scholarship. The only other one that was comparable to this was called the Queen Elizabeth Scholarship but it was only for one year and there was a lot of competition for it.

As long as I maintained a good academic standing for four years, this scholarship would cover me at the university until I got my Medical Degree (MD). This placed a heavy burden on me to work overtime to meet the requirements. Since I had no more financial worries, I could now concentrate on studying hard.

One of the courses in this first year was neuro-anatomy, the study of the brain including dissection. I was offered a job by the chief resident of neurosurgery to clean the neurosurgical laboratory every evening at the Surgical Medical Research Institute which was part of the university. My responsibility was to look after the laboratory guinea pigs and prepare the animal specimens and equipment for the residents the next day. His team was working on spinal cord regeneration following trans-section of the cord of the guinea pig.

This job gave me extra money allowing me to leave the residence and move to the nearby home of a European couple where I paid room and board. My apartment consisted of a bedroom, living room and a kitchenette. I had my meals with the others in the house and was able to have friends visit me in my apartment without any complaints from my landlady. I continued to excel in my schoolwork, and remained one of the top 10 students with high marks in my class.

One of our courses involved the neuro-anatomy lab in which we observed and carried out dissection of the brain on cadavers. This course was always on a specific day of the week. But as it turned out, my landlady who was an excellent cook had a delicacy which she served on a weekly basis that happened to be pig brain with sauerkraut.

This was the same day of the week that we attended the anatomy dissection of the brain in the autopsy room. Initially, the idea of eating cooked pig brain with sauerkraut did not bother me until one particular day it dawned on me that I was actually eating parts similar to the human brain which our class had just finished working on. My stomach revolted and I got to the point where I just could not face this meal on anatomy day.

I approached my landlady and explained the situation. She was not entirely happy about me asking for a change of menu as this had been her family routine for many years even before coming to Canada and it was her favorite meal.

She finally decided to serve me chicken while the rest of the company in the house continued to eat her delicacy. I was grateful that she did not ask me to leave her home thinking that I was unhappy with her cooking because I had developed a friendly relationship with the family and enjoyed their hospitality.

Later in the year, I was invited by a Ghanaian friend of mine who was a dental student, to join him in a suite that he was renting which had two bedrooms. It was as close to the university campus as my previous residence and we both shared the rent which helped each of us financially. We did our own cooking, sometimes with the help of our girlfriends. By this time I had made many friends and in the summer of 1963 I decided to get married.

CHAPTER SEVEN
SECOND AND THIRD YEAR OF MEDICAL SCHOOL

During my second year, which started in September of 1963, I knew I had to continue to work hard so as not to lose my scholarship. I was one of the younger students in the class and there were others better prepared academically, including two pharmacists, three students with Master of Science degrees and one student who had submitted his PhD thesis in biology. All of these factors made me realize the importance of being dedicated to my studies. I was excited one day when the professor of surgery approached me and asked if I would be interested in participating in a research project at the Surgical Medical Research Institute.

The title of the project was The Effect of Exogenously Administered D-Glucosamine Hydrochloride on the Seromucoid Fraction of Tumor-Bearing Rats.

I will try to explain this experiment as simply as possible without losing its content. The project involved the transplant of Walker 256 cancer cells from a tumor bearing rat to a non-tumor bearing rat, to see its effect on the D-Glucosamine Sulfate level of the rat with malignancy. Walker 256 cancer cells are similar to breast cancer cells in humans.

This was a difficult and time consuming project but nevertheless, it was interesting. It gave me the opportunity to get acquainted with surgical research, albeit in rats. Apparently, cancer of the breast in a rat behaves the same way as in humans.

This project was sponsored by grants from the National Cancer Institute of Canada (NCI No. 226) and the Medical Research Fund of the University of Alberta (MR No. 236). It was also sponsored by a private donation through the Vessie Heckbert Summer Research Student scholarship.

I won the University of Alberta Surgical Research prize and it was presented to me later during my graduation in 1966. This was my first opportunity to be involved in a research project at the university and encouraged me to accept another offer later on in my training. The results were accepted for publication in the Cancer Research Journal and I was proud to be a part of it.

(Reference: R.A. Macbeth and M. Akpata: Cancer Research Vol 27, Part 1, 912 to 916, 1967. The Effect of Exogenously Administered D-Glucosamine Hydrochloride on the Seromucoid Fraction of Tumor-bearing Rats.)

During my third year, I was lucky to be given the opportunity to perform another research project under the supervision of one of the surgical professors. The procedure was done under the sponsorship of the National Cancer Institute (NCI) and Hospital Research Fund. The title of the project was: 'Wound Healing in a Single Layer of Intestinal Anastomosis in Rats'.

The procedure involved the comparison of one layer of suturing for intestinal anastomosis as opposed to the regular two layers of suturing. The aim of the procedure was to find out if it was necessary to use two layers of sutures for joining the two cut ends of the bowel or if one layer would be sufficient.

The accepted procedure at that time was to close the inner lining of the bowel (mucosa) with a suture that would dissolve in a few days and then close the outside muscular layer with a non-dissolvable silk suture. Again, I was pleased to carry out this project.

Certain parameters were then measured and the findings were as follows:

• The initial bursting pressure of the two layer anastomosis was higher than that of the one layer anastomosis especially during the first 48 hours after surgery. However, the pressure gradually declined during the ensuing ten days of recording the result. It was assumed that the initial increased pressure was due to swelling of the mucosal surface of the bowel where it was joined. As the healing progressed, there was evidence of the lining of the bowel sloughing off with loss of tensile strength at the anastomotic site. Ultimately the tensile strength of the two layer anastomosis site and the bursting pressure declined.

• In the case of the one layer anastomosis, the initial bursting pressure was less than in the two layer anastomosis but the tensile strength increased due to less sloughing of the lining at the anastomotic site and the muscle behind it. The results showed that it took more tension to rupture the one layer anastomosis after a period of healing than the two layer anastomosis.

I was sponsored to present the results of this research project at the annual meeting of the Royal College of Physicians and Surgeons in Montréal in 1970 and it was well received by the entire audience. Unfortunately, this research project was not published in a surgical journal as it had been done as part of my first research.

CHAPTER EIGHT
END OF FOURTH YEAR MEDICINE

In June of 1966, I completed my training in medicine. I then started preparing for my qualification examination for the degree of Doctor of Medicine. I passed both the written and oral parts of the examination thus obtaining my MD. The next examination was for the Licentiate of the Medical Council of Canada (LMCC) and again I was happy to pass this examination.

During the oral portion of the examination for LMCC, a very interesting incident occurred. There was a foreign student who had trained in London, England and was required to update his Fellowship in Surgery (FRCS) to practice in Canada. He was a resident in the department of surgery, prominent and well-known to professors both in England and in Canada.

Because of his previous background, he was allowed to skip the written examination but still had to do the oral portion. His last name also started with the letter 'A' like mine and he was scheduled immediately after me for testing.

When I came out of the examination room, he ran to me and begged me to tell him what questions I was asked. I was relieved having completed the exam, and in a jovial manner I told him that I was asked how one would kill lice in a bed. In fact this was the actual question I was asked.

Frustrated, he admitted he knew nothing about it and wanted to know my answer to this question. I replied, "At night you place a lighted lamp at the bedside to lure any bugs and then spray the bed with a special bed bug killer."

When he finished his oral examination he came out looking excited and told me that the first thing they asked him was how he would kill lice in a bed. I expected him to relay the answer I had given him to this question. Instead, he told the examiner that you pour kerosene on the bed, light a match and throw it into the bed. I was shocked. I asked him why he said such a thing and wanted to know the examiner's response.

The professor replied; "Go on, you are just teasing me because I know you know the correct answer. It involves a process of

VNIVERSITAS · ALBERTAENSIS

HAS · LITTERAS · EDIT · VT · OMNES · AD · QVOS · EAEDEM · PERVENERINT
CERTIORES · FIANT

MICHAEL OYEWOLE AKPATA

CVM · OMNIA · QVAE · PER · STATVTA · REQVIRVNTVR · PRAESTITERIT · ET · COMPLEVERIT
TITVLO · GRADVQVE

DOCTORIS · MEDICINAE

ESSE · ADORNATVM · EIQVE · CONCESSA · OMNIA · PRIVILEGIA · ET · IVRA · HVIVS · GRADVS

CVIVS · REI · SINT · TESTIMONIO · CHIROGRAPHA · CANCELLARII
PRAESIDIS · CONCILII · GVBERNATORVM
RECTORIS · REGISTRARIIQVE · HVIVS · VNIVERSITATIS
ACCEDIT · SIGILLVM · COMMVNE

DATVM · EX · AEDIBVS · ACADEMICIS · DIE · I · MENSIS · IVNII
ANNI · POST · CHRISTVM · NATVM · MILLESIMI · NONGENTESIMI · SEXAGESIMI · SEXTI
HVIVSQVE · VNIVERSITATIS · QVINQVAGESIMI · NONI

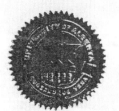

Doctor of Medicine certificate.

lighting a lamp beside the bed to attract the bugs, right? Then you spray the bed with a bug killer."

This friend of mine then said, "Yes, of course, sir." The whole crowd of students who were waiting to hear his answer all burst out laughing. Then I said, "That wasn't the answer I gave you. Lucky for you the examiner took you as the joker."

During my medical student days, even though I was immersed in my academic work, I had enough time to participate in other extracurricular activities at university. At one time I was President of the International Students Union. We used to have weekly discussions about our home backgrounds and on many occasions watched videos about our respective countries.

On the last Saturday of every month, I organized a party for all of us in the International Conference Hall with food and dancing and everyone looked forward to this event.

Another aspect of my extracurricular activity involved participating in the University Debating Society. The president of this society was Joe Clark who later became one of the Prime Ministers of Canada. I was the vice-president and I enjoyed discussing any topic of interest with the group, especially religion and politics, whether it be local and provincial, or world issues.

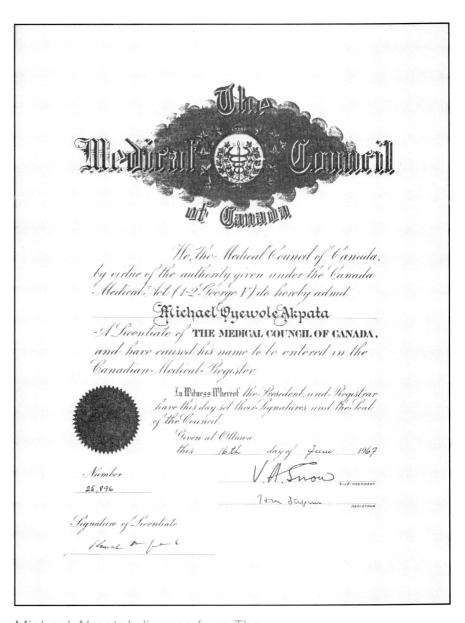

Michael Akpata's license from The Medical Council of Canada (LMCC).

Collegium Regale Medicorum et Chirurgorum Canadense

Rogante Praeside, Sociisque annuentibus, decrevit

Michael Oyewole Akpata

virum doctum,

Chirurgiae

peritum, examine rite probatum, in Societatem suam in partitionem Chirurgiae adsciscere, omniumque honorum atque privilegiorum, quibus Socii eiusdem Collegii fruuntur, participem facere.

Cuius rei nos, qui litteris hisce Collegii sigillo munitis nomina subscripsimus, testes et auctores sumus.

Datum, die XIII *mensis* III *anno* MCMLXXII

Charles G. Drake — PRAESES
J. T. MacDougall — VICE-PRAESES
James H. Graham — SECRETARIUS

Fellowship in the Royal College of Physicians and Surgeons of Canada.

CHAPTER NINE
ROTATING INTERNSHIP

I embarked on my one year of rotating internship in June of 1966 at the same institution, the University of Alberta Teaching Hospital. This was a fascinating year because I was able to learn and experience the different medical subspecialties which included general medicine, obstetrics and gynecology, general surgery and pediatrics. Also we moved into the Intern's Residence which was next to the hospital building.

Of all my rotations, general surgery was the most exciting and demanding. This included the gastroenterology portion of internal medicine. The rotating internship was so stressful that I developed an active duodenal ulcer. I was started on medication and given 10 days off duty.

But, within a few days I felt better and informed the teaching fellow in charge of interns that I was fit to return to active duty. He allowed me to return, as long as I continued to take the medicine to reduce the acid in my stomach.

During my year of internship, I had a very good friend who lived next door to me, who was also an intern. The events I'm going to discuss involved his wife who was a friend of both my wife and I. In fact, our houses were so close that we could almost shake hands across the divide through the kitchen windows.

During my rotation through obstetrics and gynecology, I did not care for obstetrics but the gynecological portion was of interest to me, possibly because it involved some surgery. I discussed my feelings with my friend and his wife one evening when we were all having dinner.

I told them that I was not interested in obstetrics because of the suffering I saw the pregnant women go through during delivery. My friend's wife said to me, "At least you are honest. Please, don't come near me in the delivery room when I'm having my baby."

She was eight months pregnant and near her time of delivery.

Early one morning, as fate would have it, she went into labor. She was rushed to hospital and transferred into the delivery room in an almost fully dilated condition. Meanwhile, her obstetrician had been called and was on his way but not yet in the building.

I was scheduled to second assist in general surgery for a bowel resection on that particular day and was scrubbing my hands to join my surgical team. Suddenly, the hospital telephone operator started paging for her obstetrician, not realizing he was still traveling to the hospital. The next announcement coming through the intercom was, "Any available obstetrician, please report to the delivery room right away."

When there was no response, the message changed to, "Any obstetrical resident or intern, please go to the delivery room."

Still nobody took the call as there was no one available. Then the final call came, "Any doctor available, please go to the delivery room."

I had just finished scrubbing when I saw the nurse in charge running towards me begging me to come immediately to help deliver a baby. I told her that I was scheduled for a case at that time as a second assistant in general surgery. After a second thought, I felt it would be wise for me to go and offer whatever help I could give.

When I entered the delivery room, to my surprise, I was confronted with my friend's wife who was crying in pain. But when she saw me, she burst out laughing.

"I don't believe this. You are actually going to be the one to deliver my baby after all."

Everyone in the room, including the anesthetist and the nurses started to laugh when they heard the story. I told my friend's wife that I would do my best for her and proceeded to deliver the baby safely without any complications.

As I began removing the placenta, her obstetrician walked in and took over the procedure. Fortunately, the mother and child did well and I was thanked by all for my part in the delivery. This experience gave us plenty to talk about later and always sparked laughter.

At the end of my rotating internship, I received my certificate of Licentiate of the Medical Council of Canada. As I was now registered with my LMCC, I was qualified as a medical doctor and able to set up my own practice. Nonetheless, I decided to apply to do my postgraduate training right away rather than leave the university environment. Besides, my wish had always been to become a surgeon. I applied for a position in the Residency Program in General Surgery and was accepted.

CHAPTER TEN
FIRST YEAR RESIDENCY PROGRAM

The residency program was a four-year course with each year titled as follows: the first year was called the Junior Assistant Resident (JAR) then the Senior Assistant Resident (SAR), the Associate Resident (AR) and the final and fourth year was called the Resident year. My first year residency in general surgery was less stressful, very refreshing and happy. I could study with no financial worries regarding school fees since we were now being paid by the university hospital.

The residents were assigned to different professors of surgery and to the Chief Resident of Surgery A or B. I developed a good relationship particularly with my own professor in Surgery A who often asked me to be second assistant for his procedures.

On one occasion, a senior professor of surgery was performing a gastroesophageal resection for a proximal gastric cancer (that is the removal of the upper part of the stomach and lower part of the esophagus for cancer). Once the upper part of the stomach and the lower esophagus had been removed, it was time for him to rejoin the esophagus to the remaining part of the stomach. He inserted a lot of sutures at this junction leaving the ends loose with the plan of tying together the two ends of each individual suture later.

Suddenly the professor yelled, "Oh no! I have an appointment in 10 minutes with the Minister of Health in my office at the hospital."

The professor looked straight at the chief resident who was the first assistant in the case and told him he would be leaving right away and that he should let Akpata finish the case. This is in spite of the fact that I was the second assistant and in my first year of the residency program.

"Yes sir", replied the chief resident to the professor. Turning to me he said, "Mike, the problem is now yours. Good luck."

The night before this surgery, I checked the operating room roster for the next day and saw this case listed for our group. I then went to the library to study the chapter on this procedure in case I was quizzed on it, either by the chief resident or the professor. So I felt somewhat comfortable to take over the case and complete it as requested.

When I looked at all the sutures that had been inserted at the junction of the stomach and the esophagus, I could not figure out which end of each suture belonged to the other. I decided to take out all the sutures and start from the beginning. I would tie each stitch as I went along before inserting another one so I would not get the ends mixed up. The procedure was a success.

The chief resident then congratulated me for what he described as, 'a fine job especially for a junior assistant resident.'

The next day when the professor saw the two of us, he asked the chief resident if I had done the job myself and he replied in the affirmative.

"Good for you Mike. I knew you could do it because I saw you reading about it in the library the night before."

He congratulated me and said that I would have a bright future in surgery if I were to continue in this manner. From then on, I always prepared for the next day's surgery by reading about it before. This was a practice I continued for any major case throughout my career.

CHAPTER ELEVEN
SECOND YEAR RESIDENCY PROGRAM

This was a tumultuous year. As well as having to learn major general surgical procedures, we also had to rotate through other surgical subspecialties which included orthopedics, cardiovascular surgery, neurosurgery, urology, and plastic surgery. This same schedule was followed during the third year.

Plastic surgery was boring for me but I was fascinated by how meticulous the work could be. Cardiovascular and neurosurgery were exciting but my primary interest was still general surgery.

As a rotating senior assistant resident, I would normally be the second assistant. During one procedure involving cardiovascular surgery, I was asked to be the first assistant even though the cardiovascular resident was present.

The case was mitral valvulotomy which involves the splitting of a heart valve blocked by scar tissue to allow blood to flow from the top section of the heart to the bottom section. The professor was an excellent surgeon and a very kind man. As the case progressed, he said to me, "Mike, you should switch from general surgery to cardiovascular surgery as your specialty. I think you'll like it and you should do very well."

I thanked him for his kind remarks and his confidence in me.

Impressed by my performance, he said, "I know the professor of cardiovascular surgery at New York University. We are very good friends, so I will call him and recommend that you be accepted as one of his residents next year."

I had no desire to give up general surgery because cancer surgery of the stomach, bowel and esophagus appealed to me more than anything else. Besides, I did not take the professor's remarks about calling his friend in New York seriously.

After we had finished the case, I went back to my apartment in the intern's residence for lunch. Unexpectedly, the telephone rang and an unfamiliar voice identified himself as the chief of cardiovascular surgery at New York University Hospital. He said he was a good friend of my cardiovascular professor who had just called him.

"If you are as good as he says you are, I will consider you for a position in my faculty residency program for next year. What do you say to that? Are you interested in this proposal?"

I really could not answer the question because I was dumbfounded and could not speak. He said, "Well do you want this position or not?" Again I hesitated. Without further discussion, he simply said, "I'll call you in one month."

Receiving a call from a professor of world repute was shocking in itself but deciding my future was also involved. My main interest was in general surgery rather than cardiovascular surgery.

The following day, I saw my professor who asked me if I had accepted his friend's offer. I told him that the call did surprise me but I needed some time to think about it. He was very disappointed that I did not accept his offer.

Exactly one month to the day, while I was again having lunch at the intern's residence, I received a call from the same professor asking me if I had made a decision regarding his offer. He noticed my vacillation and said, "Mike, goodbye" and hung up the phone.

CHAPTER TWELVE
ASSOCIATE RESIDENT YEAR

As an associate resident, my role was that of the first assistant and I was now in a position to be responsible for performing numerous procedures. As in the previous year, I was still expected to rotate through certain subspecialties. I also decided to accept any offer to carry out surgical research at the Surgical Medical Research Institute regarding intestinal surgery, but there was none on the horizon. The hours of work were strenuous but we accomplished and learned a lot.

During my rotation in plastic surgery, there was an unusual incident which was sad but somewhat humorous.

This was a case of a woman in her forties and her involvement with two male friends. She had had a relationship for a number of years with an older man who was a very successful pig farmer, but he was not willing to get married. He knew the lady very well over the years and still had a key to her house. They eventually broke off their relationship and she soon befriended another man much younger in his mid-thirties.

One evening the lady and the young man went to a local bar which she had frequented for years with her ex-boyfriend. After they both had quite a few alcoholic drinks, she invited the young man back to her house.

The young man had apparently fallen asleep on the living room couch while the lady was sleeping in her bedroom. Someone quietly opened the door to the house and with great accuracy and precision made a cut over the young man's scrotum and surgically removed his testicles. It was amazing that he was able to carry out this procedure and slip out of the house before the man was awake.

This poor young man woke up to see that he was bleeding profusely and became terrified. He started screaming and woke up the girlfriend who immediately rushed him to a nearby hospital emergency department.

I was the rotating associate resident on call for plastic surgery that evening. We immediately started resuscitative measures, cross-matched him for blood and rushed him into the operating room. I made an urgent call for help to the professor of plastic surgery and he was in the operating room with me in no time.

We evacuated numerous blood clots from the scrotum through a small extension of the incision the assailant had previously made. We were in the process of tying off all the bleeding vessels when a police officer ran into the emergency department.

He said to the nurse in charge, "When we went to investigate this incident, we found these two round objects on the floor and we placed them in a plastic bag."

He handed the bag to the nurse and after a quick look, she rushed into the operating room. In that bag were the patient's two testicles! That was when we realized that this man had been castrated.

Fortunately, our patient did well post surgically and his vital signs remained stable. This incident happened a day before I finished my rotation in plastic surgery. I was happy to return to my general surgical rotation.

Over the years I had taken a special interest in surgery of the pancreas, principally because the professor who was doing these procedures was affable and willing to teach anyone who showed interest in this particular area of general surgery. His specialty was hepatobiliary and pancreatic surgery which involves diseases of the liver, pancreas, gallbladder and bile ducts.

One day, this professor asked me to take over a surgical case called Whipple's procedure. This involves the removal of part of the pancreas, part of the stomach and the first portion of the small bowel to treat cancer of the head of the pancreas. This tedious procedure requires about eight hours of surgery.

"Mike this is your case today and I know you can do it. Of course, I shall be with you throughout to make sure you do not screw up, ha, ha, ha!"

I was honored and gratified by the confidence he expressed in allowing me to do this procedure. Normally, only a fourth year resident would have this opportunity.

The patient was a healthy 52-year-old man with no previous family history of cancer of the pancreas and preoperative workup did not show any evidence of the tumor spreading. The tumor was found during a routine workup because he had complained of pain in the abdomen radiating to the back. He did not show any sign of weight loss, low hemoglobin or jaundice which meant that it was probably in the early stages.

With meticulous dissection, I was able to remove the head and neck of the pancreas together with the duodenum and the lower part of the stomach. Examination of the abdomen showed no evidence of the disease spreading.

The professor was obviously pleased with my work and confirmed it when he said to me, "Well done, now it is time for you to put the rest of these organs back together which will not be easy."

I was shocked again thinking he was going to take over from me at this point to finish the case. Instead, I had to perform the rest of the procedure. After I closed the abdomen, the patient was transferred into the general surgical intensive care unit.

This became my greatest achievement up to this point in my career.

The patient was also followed by the professor and during one of our monthly clinical pathology conferences, he discussed this case. I was elated to hear him say, "Mike did this case in my presence with flair!"

CHAPTER THIRTEEN
FOURTH YEAR RESIDENCY

During that final year, two of us were chosen to be the chief residents. The general surgical department was divided into two sections - Surgery A and Surgery B. Each section had a chief resident in charge of running the operating room for his own section. I was appointed chief resident for Surgical Group A.

Part of my job was to book the cases for the surgical professors in our group. I had the opportunity to perform Whipple's procedures, gastrectomy (removal of part or all of the stomach), large and small bowel resection, removal of the spleen, appendix, gallbladder and varicose veins of the legs.

There was an interesting case during my chief residency year when I overstepped my bounds. I was the first assistant in a difficult open gallbladder surgery being done by one of the professors on our team. He was concerned that there were stones in the common duct which connects the neck of the gallbladder to the portion of the small bowel called the duodenum. If there were stones present, they would have to be removed to prevent blockage of the duct and create further complications.

Back then, there was no ultrasound or CT Scan to help visualize the stones before surgery and the abdominal x-rays were not accurate enough to show whether common duct stones were present. The professor decided to do what we call an intra-operative cholangiogram.

This involves the injection of dye into the cystic duct followed by x-rays while the patient is still asleep on the operating table. Once the films were hung on the view box, the professor was able to review them and I could hear him say that there were no stones in the common duct.

At this point, I immediately removed the gallbladder myself. When the professor arrived back at his spot to continue the surgery, he was shocked to find that the gallbladder had been removed and I could see that he was quite upset.

Then he said to me, "Well, Dr. Smart Ass, you might as well finish the rest of the procedure."

I was shaking in my boots because I knew I should not have completed his case. So I apologized and never again overstepped my bounds with this professor.

Finally, while completing my chief residency year, there was an intern who was not particularly interested in surgery and was always absent from the operating room during his rotation in general surgery.

He did not like to scrub for any surgical procedure and had never even seen an appendectomy (removal of appendix), let alone do one on his own under the guidance of the resident. He deliberately disappeared whenever there was a case in which he was supposed to participate.

Then one day he complained to the professor of surgery that he had not had the opportunity to do any procedure in general surgery on his own during his rotation.

Shortly after, the situation presented itself for him to be invited into the operating room for removal of an infected appendix. I was the chief resident in charge and took the opportunity to call this intern to come and assist me.

His answer was, "Thank you, Mike, I don't mind reading about it but I am not really interested in hands-on surgery. My preference is psychiatry."

I was shocked to hear this from an intern who had complained to the professor a few days before that he was denied the opportunity to perform any minor surgery in the operating room. At the end of his rotational internship, he did enroll to become a psychiatrist.

In June of 1971, I had completed my residency year in general surgery and was ready to sit for my fellowship examination. This involved both a written and an oral section. I passed the written section and was now preparing for the orals in September, at Montréal General Hospital.

The professors felt we should have mock orals in preparation for this day. They would ask questions of each resident and later it would be discussed by the entire group.

During one of those question and answer periods, one of the professors asked me to describe a particular procedure involving the anatomy of the groin. I gave my answer in great detail, and the next thing I heard from the professor was "BS."

I was shocked and upset by his comment. He said I should have replied in a simpler manner instead of expanding my answer as I did. When he asked the members of the audience to comment on my answer, there was utter silence in the room. No one was willing to give an opinion because they thought the professor and I were both right. It was a matter of me being too specific.

However, just before the oral examination, the professor announced to the group, "By the way, Mike was correct in his lengthy response to my question a few days ago." He then wished us good luck in our forthcoming trip to Montreal.

I was relieved that I was successful in my oral exam. It had been a long journey from my first days of entering the doors of the University of Alberta to becoming a doctor. I was grateful for the training offered to me and my thanks go to the professors who mentored me throughout the years. I also thank God for blessing me with the tolerance and strength to undergo eleven years of university training obtaining my Fellowship in General Surgery, FRCS (C).

CHAPTER FOURTEEN
APPOINTMENT AS A TEACHING FELLOW

Although I was now a full-fledged general surgeon in good standing at the University of Alberta, my ultimate goal was to become a general surgical oncologist. But, I had to be accepted into one of the well-known cancer clinic hospitals either in Canada or the United States. In the meantime, I was looking forward to my job as a Teaching Fellow to gain additional experience before embarking on my career.

This new position would allow me to function as a quasi assistant professor in the department of general surgery. My role was to look after patients not attached to any surgeon both electively and on an emergency basis. I was no longer under the supervision of a professor of surgery and part of my job included the teaching of medical students and some residents up to the senior assistant level. I was able to perform any major or minor surgical procedure that came my way and it was my job to follow the patients until they were discharged home. It was quite an opportunity to improve my surgical expertise.

This fellowship position was for one year. Prior to its termination, I had to make some important decisions regarding my future life plans. I had many choices in my mind, including the following:

• Return to Nigeria either to join the University Hospital in Lagos or to set up my own private practice. I was reluctant to go back home at this time as the country was under a military dictatorship.

• Apply for an Oregon license to set up practice in Portland, Oregon. Luckily my application for this license was accepted and I had offers from two hospitals to join their staff. But, I really wanted to leave the cold weather of the west and thought the East Coast of either Canada or United States might be a better option. As a back-up plan, I paid the annual dues to maintain my Oregon license.

• Apply for training in surgical oncology at Memorial Sloan Kettering Institute in New York City as I had a strong interest in cancer surgery. I had an informal interview with the Institute and they were quite receptive to having me join their program. I was told that I would have to do one year of Radiology Oncology first, preferably at the University of London Health Sciences in London, Ontario, before my application would be considered for the following year of surgical oncology training. I was pleased but when I thought about it carefully, I realized that I would be very restricted as to

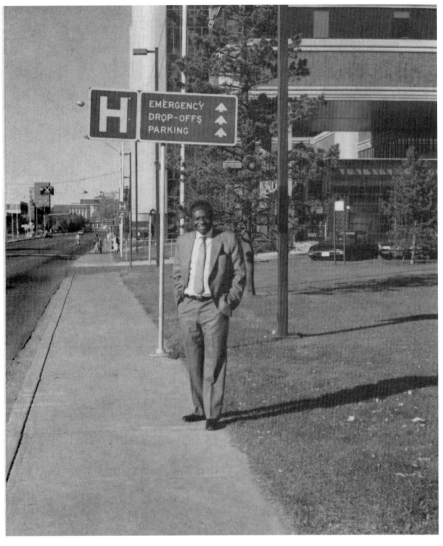

Dr. Michael Akpata was appointed as a teaching fellow for one year at the University of Alberta Hospital.

where I could work if I did only cancer surgery.

While I was debating all my options, I received an unexpected call from a classmate who was now an orthopedic surgeon wanting me to join him in a clinic in Wetaskiwin, near Edmonton. He suggested that this would be an opportunity for me to begin a practice and be paid while I deliberated on my future plans.

After one year of private practice with my friend, I had an offer from a clinical group in Red Deer, Alberta to join them as their surgeon. This contract was supposed to last one year but before I knew it I had completed four years there.

I thoroughly enjoyed being the surgeon for this clinic but I thought it was time for me to finally set up my own independent surgical practice and leave the cold west.

CHAPTER FIFTEEN
APPLICATION TO GRACE HOSPITAL TORONTO

There were several choices of hospitals where I could apply for privileges to practice surgery in Toronto. However, the only one which had adequate bed facilities was Grace Hospital where my application was accepted. Shortly after I had started practicing, the administration decided that the hospital would be converted to only obstetrics and gynecology.

I was surprised and quite disappointed because I was just getting settled. The administrator told the surgeons at the hospital that we should look around for any other Grace Hospital in Ontario and that he would recommend us for privileges in any one we chose.

I visited several of the Grace Hospitals including the ones at Oakville and Ottawa. The granting of hospital privileges was not a problem but the facilities for a proper surgical practice were grossly limited.

I liked the Oakville site because of its close proximity to Toronto but after I spoke to the administration, I was told that the bed situation was very critical and that at the most I would be assigned only one bed per week. I could not imagine how an active surgeon could function on such a limited bed allocation.

It would mean that the bulk of my surgery would have to be day surgery not requiring an overnight stay and the number of major surgical cases that I could do would be very restricted.

Grace Hospital in Ottawa was appealing because besides it being the capital of the country, I would be in close proximity to the daily political situations as politics is one of my special interests. But again, there were inadequate beds available to new members of the surgical staff.

During my visit to Ottawa, I was informed by one of the surgeons that my best option was to go to Windsor because he had heard that additional surgeons were required there and also that there were three other hospitals to choose from. I thanked him and decided to take his advice to explore the facilities in Windsor.

CHAPTER SIXTEEN
MOVE TO WINDSOR

On a beautiful sunny day during the summer, a friend and I decided to drive from Toronto to Windsor. This was my first trip to southwestern Ontario. Upon our arrival in London, we spent a few hours browsing around the city and the University Hospital campus before we continued on to Windsor. At about 20 km outside the city, I could see the skyline which looked very enticing and I began to get quite excited about choosing Windsor as my place of work and residence. But, when we arrived in the downtown area it became obvious that the skyline I was admiring was actually that of Detroit and not Windsor. Nevertheless, the trip down Riverside Drive overlooking the Renaissance Center was very pleasant.

I then decided to apply to Grace Hospital for admitting privileges in general surgery and endoscopy. The only question that crossed my mind for the first time since I had arrived in Canada was whether Windsor was cosmopolitan and open-minded enough to accept me as a foreigner of different racial background to become one of their surgeons.

Up to this point living in Canada, I had never worried about not being accepted based on my race. Possibly because I was now going to be competing with other surgeons, and before I had been working in a group practice in smaller towns, this concern arose. I decided to press on with my plans.

The following day, I made a call to the hospital and asked for an appointment with the chairman of the credentials committee to present my papers from Grace Hospital in Toronto. They were already aware of the plans to change the mandate of the Toronto Hospital branch and therefore I was granted privileges.

Shortly after, I ran into Dr. Joseph Galiwango who was a pediatrician from Uganda. Happy to see me move to Windsor, he suggested that I should also apply for privileges in the other three hospitals; Windsor Western, Metropolitan and Hôtel Dieu. As suggested, I sent my applications to these three places and after interviews, I was granted admitting privileges to all of them.

Unlike the hospitals in Oakville and Ottawa, no mention was made to me about bed shortages or allocations in any of these four hospitals. I now felt that I had made the right decision and was very comfortable in moving my family to Windsor to set up my surgical practice.

Having privileges in all four hospitals, it became imperative that I find a centrally located place to set up my office practice. Dr. Galiwango was available to guide me since I had no prior knowledge of the city. His office was located at the 700 Tecumseh Road complex and he offered me the opportunity of sharing his office space until I found a place of my own.

I didn't think the combination of pediatrician and general surgeon in one location was a good idea so I thanked him and declined the offer.

He introduced me to the director of the Windsor Health Center and I enquired if there was any office space available. I was told that the main Tecumseh Road complex was filled but there was a warehouse facility in the empty 630 building which could be converted into office space.

After exploring other options in the city, I saw the advantage of being close to referring physicians from the 700 building and eventually went back to negotiate a price. This same director arranged for my office to be constructed which would consist of two examination rooms, a private office, waiting room and a secretary's area. I purchased all the necessary furniture, medical equipment and supplies that I would need for my work.

While all the construction was being done, I commuted back and forth to Toronto by rail in order to be with my family. I also did locums in various areas of northern Ontario communities until I was ready to make the move to Windsor.

Once all the necessary documents for my office had been signed, the building manager took me to the former Bank of Montréal building on Riverside Drive and introduced me to the bank manager who set up a business account for me.

While we were conducting these transactions, the bank manager asked if I was interested in buying his house which actually belonged to the bank. He was being transferred to another city and the new manager already had purchased a place of residence for himself. I was happy to have this opportunity to purchase a beautiful home in South Windsor.

Once this transaction was completed, all the arrangements were finally made to bring my family to our new home.

The business manager of the medical complex also took me to a friend of his who owned a Volvo dealership where I was able to purchase a car. When I look back on this time, I realize how helpful he was in all aspects.

By the end of December 1979, I had hired a secretary, a middle-aged lady whose previous experience in another doctor's office was a great asset in setting up my office. I placed an announcement in the Windsor Star and was now ready to embark on my practice of general surgery and endoscopy. When my family arrived in Windsor, my three children were enrolled at the Central Public School, a few blocks away from our house.

CHAPTER SEVENTEEN
BEGINNING MY PRACTICE

In those days, the referring physician always assisted on the surgery for his own patients and so was made aware of the time, date and place of the surgery so that he would be available. However, on one occasion, the family doctor was assisting in another hospital so the surgeon asked if I would be willing to assist him. I saw an opportunity to expose myself to the other surgeons in the operating room and I was quite willing to assist them whenever they ran into this problem, day or night.

Gradually my referral pattern increased when the family physicians realized that I was willing to help them out when they were not available. I developed a friendly relationship with most of them and on several occasions we had the opportunity to attend a sponsored dinner meeting together. This gave the family physicians the chance outside of surgery and to get to know my type of personality. As time went on, I continued to get more referrals from both the younger and the more established physicians.

When I first arrived in town, there was no organized pattern of surgical emergency coverage in the four hospitals as there is now. Bearing in mind that most of us had privileges in all four hospitals, it was our expected duty to cover emergency services in all of them.

This made it very strenuous for physicians and surgeons alike. Far more difficult and demanding was the fact that once a family physician had chosen a particular surgeon for his elective cases, it was expected that this same surgeon would cover the emergency cases in any of the hospitals irrespective of the time of day or night and including weekends and holidays. As my practice increased in volume, so did my need to attend the four emergency departments to look after my family physician's patients.

This put great stress on my life as I was the newest general surgeon in town and had to develop a reputation for being able, reliable and available in order to get referrals.

On a snowy December evening, one of the family physicians who usually referred all of his cases to another particular surgeon had one of his patients show up in the emergency department in septic shock from intestinal perforation. The nurse in charge called the physician to notify him of his patient's critical condition. He told her to notify his regular referring surgeon who as it turned out was not available. On this latest notification, he then said, "Try Dr. Akpata. He is always available."

It was Christmas Eve and I was on my way to the church service, but I felt obligated to see this patient and so I changed my plans. When I arrived at the emergency department, I saw the patient was indeed in septic shock with a very low blood pressure.

X-rays showed free air in the abdomen and dilated loops of bowel with some areas of ischemia (inadequate blood supply). I examined the patient and realizing the seriousness of the situation, had him transferred directly into the operating room for surgery. I discussed my concern with his wife, and the possible consequences of the surgery. She was quite willing to sign the hospital consent.

Once the abdomen was open, I was able to locate the site where the perforation had occurred and had to remove a portion of the bowel. The abdominal cavity was grossly infected so I could not rejoin the two ends of the bowel. I gave this patient a temporary colostomy and then transferred him into the intensive care unit with heavy doses of antibiotics and several blood transfusions.

After surgery, the patient did well but it took many days to bring him back to the stage that he was able to function normally. I followed him until he was discharged home and arranged to see him in my office for reassessment. Six months later, this patient underwent his final surgery to reattach the ends of the bowel and after follow up he was returned to the care of his regular family doctor.

I was glad that the patient had survived his ordeal. Both he and his family were grateful and thanked me for saving his life. I told them they should thank God as I was only an instrument in the process.

Shortly after, it became obvious that the surgical department had to come up with a plan to set up a roster with a fair distribution of names and dates to cover each of the four hospitals on a regular basis. This new method has worked effectively for many years.

I was willing to accept referrals from physicians to see patients for office, hospital or emergency surgical consultations regardless of the severity of their problems. This increased my workload to the extent that sometimes I was in the hospital up to 14 hours a day and the complexity of the cases I was dealing with increased with time. There were many times when my office consultations were postponed because of delays in the operating room or additional emergency cases.

I was able to book some surgeries at Hôtel Dieu but the majority of my work was being done at Windsor Western as they had more operating room time available.

During the time from my arrival in Windsor to the early 1990's, there was not a qualified Intensivist in any of the hospitals. For example, at Windsor Western, Dr. Ismail Peer and I managed most of the patients in the intensive care unit.

To maintain and improve my skills, I attended intensive care courses every year both in Canada and the United States including the University of Michigan Medical School and the University of Southern California.

During the first 10 years of practice, the pace of my work in Windsor bordered on excessive. It was not unusual for me to spend up to 100 hours a week on my job including the time I spent during the weekends in the office catching up on dictations and accumulating paperwork. In most instances I was in the hospital up to 8 pm daily. This was a matter of choice but I was young and strong and I felt obliged to check on my patient's progress before going home. I was also on call for surgical emergencies for one of the hospitals almost daily.

Once I had a serious emergency case involving a young man about 40 years old who had had an altercation with two other men over his failure to pay for a drug deal.

He was violently beaten to near death by his assailants with metal rods, punches and kicks. Upon arrival at the emergency department, his vital signs were unstable. Complete resuscitative measures were started including insertion of an intravenous line for fluids, Foley catheter into his bladder and nasogastric tube into the stomach for suction. He was quickly transferred into the operating room for surgery. X-rays were suspicious for a possible ruptured spleen.

When I opened the abdomen, I found that his spleen had been shattered into fragments and he was bleeding profusely. It was urgent that I clamp off the main vessel feeding the spleen as soon as possible and then remove the fragmented parts to stop the flow of blood.

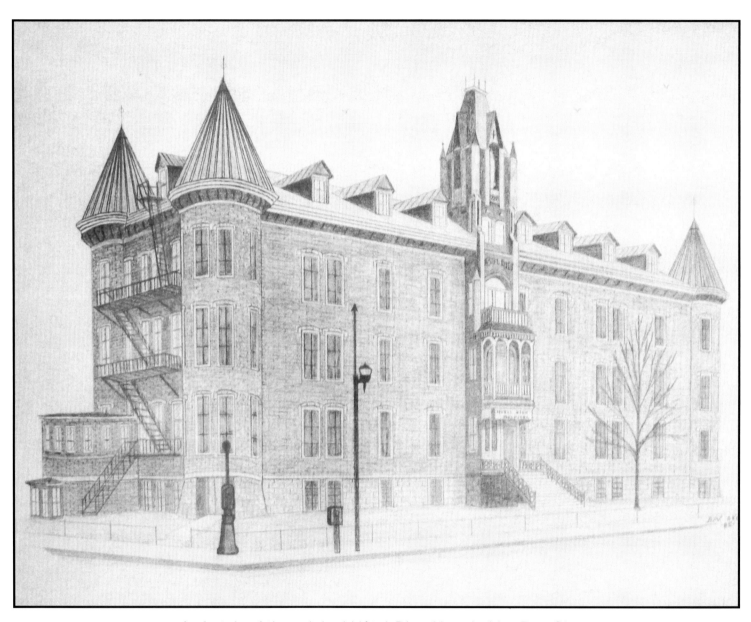

A sketch of the original Hôtel-Dieu Hospital by Bev Oke.

The anesthetist worked feverishly at his end to keep the patient stable with blood transfusions, intravenous fluids and various drugs to elevate his blood pressure. This finally gave me the opportunity to explore the abdomen further to be sure that no other injuries especially lacerations to the bowel were present.

There were a few areas in the loops of bowel requiring suturing before the abdomen could be washed out with copious amounts of saline. Drainage tubes were inserted and connected to suction machines in order to prevent any further collection of fluid in the abdomen. The abdomen was then closed and the patient was transferred to the intensive care unit for management. He was receiving drugs through the intravenous line to prevent infection and was also kept on a ventilator to help him breathe.

He had survived only the first crisis on his road to recovery.

Three days later, he was visited by a man who claimed to be his friend. The nurse stepped out of the area for a short time to allow them to visit privately. Unknown to any staff member, this friend was actually one of his assailants.

The visitor pulled out the patient's nasogastric tube, poured the water from a flower vase over his face leaving the flowers sticking out of his mouth and quickly disappeared.

Hearing the moaning noises coming from the patient's room, the nurse returned and was shocked to see the sight before her. She immediately pulled out the flowers and suctioned the patient's mouth to clear all the fluid and debris. The police were contacted and after a lengthy period of recovery, the patient was willing to identify the person who had carried out this attack.

Later on that evening, I was paged through the hospital intercom. I picked up the telephone to answer the call and before I even had a chance to speak, a male voice said, "If Mr. X survives, you are dead" and hung up.

We spoke with the police officer at the patient's doorway who reassured me that I would be safe and should not worry. I was not totally comforted by these words and had a few sleepless nights.

After two weeks of hospital stay, the patient was discharged with an appointment to see me in my office for follow up. As for the threat to my life, the police apprehended the suspect and among other things, he was charged for uttering a death threat against me.

CHAPTER EIGHTEEN
HÔTEL DIEU 100 YEAR ANNIVERSARY

Shortly after my arrival in town, it was almost time for Hôtel Dieu to celebrate its hundred year anniversary. I had developed a good relationship with the administrative staff, including the Chief Executive Offi-

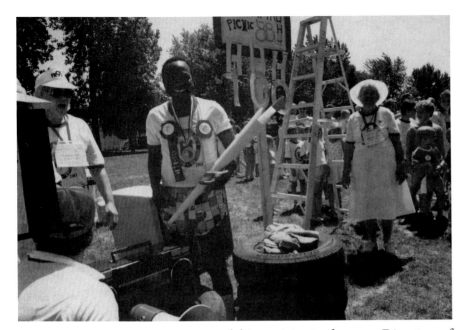

Michael accepting the torch during the celebration of the 100 year anniversary of Hôtel-Dieu Hospital at Mic Mac park.

cer and his assistant who was Director of Nursing. One day in 1988, just prior to the planned celebration at Mic Mac park, I was approached to be the torch bearer for the event. I agreed to accept the position.

The following is a brief summary of the history of Hôtel Dieu obtained from the hospital web site.

The hospital was officially founded in the fall of 1888. Dean T. Wagner, the pastor of St. Alphonsus church at that time was concerned about the poor black people who had migrated from the southern United States to the Windsor area and were members of the parish. Wagner felt that the children of the new immigrants were neglected by the local people in that they were not allowed to attend white schools and many were orphaned.

He wanted to organize a mission for black people but this required funding.

After receiving permission from the Bishop, he sent letters asking for donations. One of these letters reached the Religious Hospitallers of St. Joseph in Montréal. The Mother Superior responded by saying that if a hospital was built in Windsor, they would come and help him in his endeavor. There had been talk of building a hospital but there was a lack of interest as well as the lack of funds to operate it. After discussions with city officials and the Religious Hospitallers, six vacant lots on Ouellette Avenue were purchased. On September 14, 1888, five sisters arrived from Montréal to look after the sick and the poor with a secondary objective of teaching black children.

Dean Wagner was eventually responsible for the first hospital being built in Windsor.

During the first year, 126 patients were admitted into the hospital. The first surgical operation was performed in 1890 on a homemade operating table. The first ambulance in Windsor was obtained in 1891 at a cost of $450. Over the years, additional beds were added as needed until in 1962 the capacity reached 450 beds.

In 1907, a School of Nursing was opened within the hospital to provide facilities for the education and training of nurses. In 1945, because of an increase in the need for nurses, the Jeanne Mance School of Nursing was opened as a live-in residence for nursing students. It had to close in 1973 when the gov-

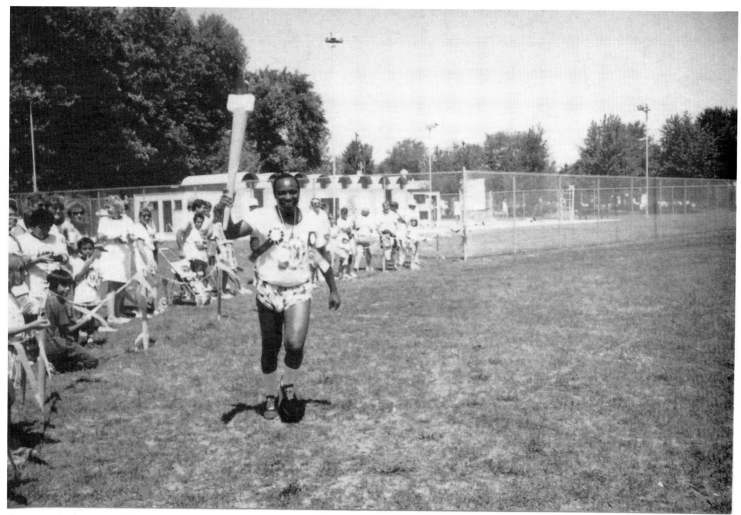
As torch bearer, Michael introduces the torch to the crowd.

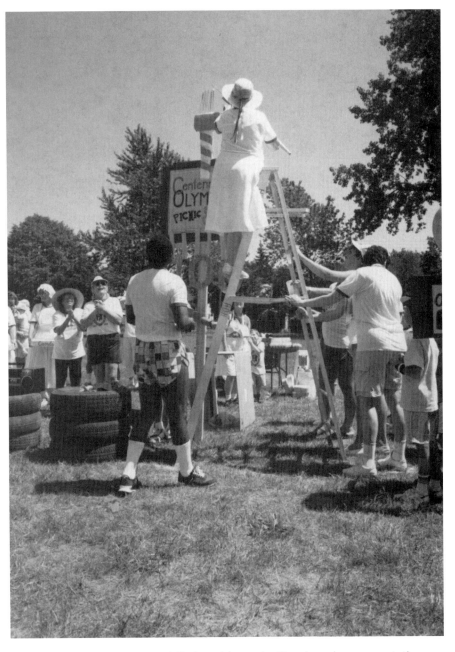

Michael hands the torch over at the end of the race.

ernment decided that all training for nurses should be done in community colleges. From 1907 to 1973, more than 1,868 nurses graduated from the school of nursing.

The nuns were still active and efficient in the running of the hospital but also directly involved in the centennial celebration. Mic Mac park was full of members of hospital staff including nurses, nuns and members of the administration. A wooden podium about eight feet high with steps leading to the top was positioned in the park. A large candle was hoisted on the top.

With torch in hand, I ran around the park where all those present were clapping and cheering.

Having been used to distance running, this was not a strenuous job for me. At one point, one of the nurses threw flower petals in front of me in a festive manner.

Once I got to the site of the wooden podium, I handed the torch over to one of the nuns waiting at the foot of the steps. She carefully climbed to the top and lit the candle.

Everyone in the audience clapped as she came down and handed the flaming torch back to me. Then I ran a short distance to allow people present to take pictures before the flame was extinguished. It was a remarkable event, bringing together the entire hospital staff to socialize and celebrate the hundred year anniversary.

CHAPTER NINETEEN
BEGINNING OF NEW PROCEDURES

When I first arrived in Windsor, the only source of venous access for surgery was through the peripheral vein on the wrist. This was usually inserted by the anesthetist and was the route used for blood and fluid infusions. It was also used for the injection of antibiotics during or after surgery.

However it was not useful for measuring any problems involving the functioning of the heart, lungs and the systemic circulation of the body unlike the new method of intravenous insertion called the central venous catheter.

On one occasion, I saw an advertisement for an intensive care course including the insertion of this catheter for the management of critically ill patients at the University of Michigan, in Ann Arbor. I registered for this course as did my colleague, Dr. Peer, since the two of us were looking after the intensive care patients at Windsor Western.

The three most central routes of insertion were through the femoral vein, that is the large vein in the groin, the internal jugular vein in the neck and the subclavian vein which is close to the edge of the clavicle. This last one was the one used most often at many major medical centers for critically ill patients.

When I returned from the course, I gave tutorials to the nurses and any interested physicians regarding the use of this catheter and how to insert it.

The anesthetists and I at Windsor Western decided to make it our priority to insert this subclavian catheter pre-operatively in all major surgical cases making it possible to measure more parameters. It was a lifesaver.

This enabled us to monitor the need to increase or decrease a patient's fluid level, easily take multiple blood samples and give nutritional feedings to enhance the recovery of the patient.

Initially, I thought this procedure would be difficult as it is imperative to avoid puncturing the artery and lung, injuring the surrounding tissues. As time went on, I developed the ability to do it with ease.

On many occasions either Dr. Peer or I was contacted to perform this procedure at Grace Hospital.

Another avenue I was exploring was the use of laser as a new innovation in surgery.

Laser is an acronym for 'light amplification by stimulated emission of radiation' and is a form of light.

Laser light differs from ordinary light in that it travels in a single direction that consists of only one wavelength. It converts light energy to heat. The laser beam can be directed to a very specific area without damaging surrounding tissue.

Laser produces a dryer surgical field, decreases pain, scarring and swelling leading to a quicker recovery and getting the patient home and back to work sooner.

Since the surgery time is shortened, there has been a shift to more outpatient and local anesthesia procedures. These are only a handful of the advantages of laser surgery.

There are many types of lasers that exist but carbon dioxide is the one I used the most.

In December of 1988, I felt that this new innovation of laser would be useful in the field of general surgery. It was being heralded in surgical literature as a better way of managing many surgical procedures rather than the use of electrocautery. In order to bring this idea to fruition, hospital administration would have to provide the necessary laser equipment. Secondly, the surgeons of different subspecialties would have to be trained in the appropriate use of this sophisticated equipment.

To underline the need for laser surgery in our hospital, I spoke with David Baker, the assistant CEO at Hôtel Dieu, regarding the purchase of laser equipment. He was reluctant to grant my request because of maintenance costs and the fact that only a few other surgeons were interested or trained in this procedure. I informed him that I was willing to go for training. He assured me that if I took this step, he would reconsider his decision.

Luckily, I was supported by Dr. Julius Schumacher, a member of the obstetrics and gynecology department, who felt that a laser machine would be an asset to the hospital.

I registered for a one week course in laser surgery at the University of Los Angeles, California which was financially exorbitant but the extent of the teaching made it worthwhile.

When I returned from my training, the assistant CEO was quite receptive to my request and consequently bought a CO_2 laser machine. A select group of nurses were trained in all of the safety aspects of laser use.

I started using laser for the removal of hemorrhoids, treatment of anal fissures and fistulae and the treatment of large anal warts, (Condylomata acuminata) which if left untreated, can sometimes become cancer of the anus.

I also used laser for the treatment of inoperable cancer of the ano-rectum as a palliative measure, in this case for a patient too old and medically unfit for major surgery. This machine was also used for gynecological and ENT (ear, nose and throat) procedures.

Surgical stapling which was introduced in the 1980s was a huge advancement to general surgery in particular. Before, there was very limited use of stapling devices and all work was done by hand suturing. Surgical stapling devices are used to reattach the two ends of a bowel which has been cut to remove a tumor.

In 1989, the Auto Suture Company of Canada arranged a dinner presentation and all interested surgeons were invited to attend and have an opportunity to discuss this new method of surgical stapling in both general and thoracic surgery.

Following this, Dr. Richard Anderson and I were invited by the company to attend a course at Toronto Western Hospital. We were both very delighted and agreed to participate in this innovative and worthwhile course at no cost to us.

There were also many candidates present from Toronto and the University of Western Ontario, in London. The course was directed by certified technicians of the Auto Suture Company in the application and handling of the devices. We were taught the use of straight, curved and circular stapling devices.

Initially, on our arrival back to Windsor, the equipment was provided by the company as well as a technician to be present in the operating room to guide us. Once we became adept in the use of the different types of stapling appliances, the hospitals purchased the necessary equipment.

At that time, I was working mostly at Windsor Western and occasionally at Hôtel Dieu.

These stapling devices made procedures easier and faster resulting in fewer complications, including bleeding and anastomotic leaks. Initially, using this stapling technique was a rarity but now it is the preferred method for many different surgical procedures and has been a great benefit to our patients. The hospitals also saw the benefit of these devices and therefore had no reluctance in purchasing them.

CHAPTER TWENTY
AGE OF LAPAROSCOPY

Laparoscopy or 'key-hole surgery' is a minimally invasive procedure and the latest surgical innovation. It involves the use of a fiber-optic scope with an attached camera and a light source which magnifies the structures to be examined two to seven times the size. These images are then projected on a television screen placed in front of the surgeon for easy visualization.

For abdominal surgery, besides using the fiber-optic scope, there are numerous instruments that can be inserted into the abdomen through very tiny holes called trocar insertion sites. These instruments are used to carry out the operation without requiring a large incision in the abdomen.

As far back as 1976, this method was designed and used in gynecological surgery and it was not until 1987 when it was first used in general surgery.

The first gallbladder surgery done laparoscopically was carried out by Dr. Philippe Mouret and his associates in Lyon, France.

It was introduced to the United States in 1988 and then to Canada at about the same time.

In 1990, after a lot of investigative reading on this new advancement in general surgery, I decided that I would like to learn it myself.

Because I had previously been encouraged by a technician from the Auto Suture Company, I approached them to sponsor me for this course. Within a few days, I received a letter from Dr. Murray Girotti, Professor and Chief of Surgery at Victoria Hospital, London.

I had been accepted as part of the first team of surgeons in Southwestern Ontario to be trained in laparoscopic cholecystectomy, the removal of the gallbladder.

As my sponsor, the Auto Suture Company covered all of my costs for the early November course at Victoria Hospital campus. Dr. Anderson, I learned later, was also included for this course.

The course began with an introduction and history of laparoscopy, a media film presentation and a discussion of the possible complications. We were then introduced to the different types of instruments and their use including the laparoscope with the attached camera, the trocars and the intra-abdominal insufflator.

Each surgeon then participated in a pig animal lab doing a minimum of three surgeries. During each case one of us acted as a surgeon and a second one as the assistant and camera man. The second step involved the observation of live human cases by specialists in this field.

After learning this procedure for two days, I received my certificate confirming my training in laparoscopic cholecystectomy. This course confirmed in my mind that this was the direction I wanted to pursue. I could definitely see the benefit especially for patients who would normally have spent up to a week in hospital plus an extended recovery time at home.

After this course, I decided to further my abilities with more in-depth training. Dr. Demetrius Litwin, Professor of Laparoscopic Surgery, at Saskatoon City Hospital was recommended to me and fortunately, he accepted my request for additional training. He informed me that first, I had to apply for and obtain a temporary license from the College of Physicians and Surgeons of Saskatchewan since I was from Ontario and not a practicing surgeon in that province.

I obtained a letter that I was in good standing with the College of Physicians and Surgeons of Ontario and with CMPA (Canadian Medical Protective Association) which covers all surgeons in Canada. I also had to commit to pay the sum of $1000 per day to the Saskatoon City Hospital and $50 to their College for its temporary license.

Once I fulfilled all these requirements, I underwent intensive training under Dr. Litwin who allowed me to assist as well as perform as many laparoscopic gallbladder cases as were available under his supervision. This training, starting on February 20, 1991, lasted three days. I was given a certificate to confirm the fact that I was now well qualified to start practicing laparoscopic cholecystectomy on my own.

After coming back to Windsor, I approached Carol Gagnon, Head of the Operating Room and Andrea Wogan, Purchasing Agent at Windsor Western in regards to obtaining the equipment needed for laparoscopic gallbladder surgery.

Open surgery was quite painful with accompanying nausea and a lengthy stay in hospital due to the size of the incision. With laparoscopic surgery, pain was minimal, hospital stay decreased to one night and patients could return to work sooner. The advantages by far outweighed the disadvantages.

The administrators saw the cost savings with a decreased hospital stay resulting in a faster turnover of bed space.

The Auto Suture Company was willing to provide disposable instruments for a period of time once the hospital purchased the basic camera, screen and insufflator. They also were willing to provide teaching to the nursing staff in regards to the care and running of the equipment. I also participated in teaching them the surgical aspect of the procedure.

Shortly after, a few of my colleagues also took the course as they realized that this

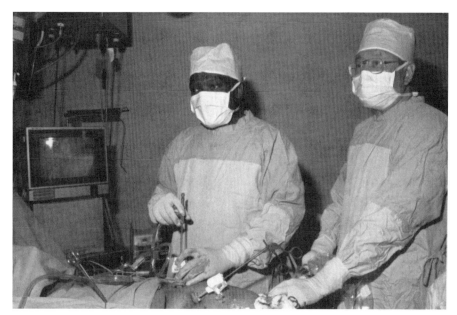
Dr. Akpata [left] is assisted by Dr. John Yee while performing laparoscopic surgery at Windsor Western Hospital.

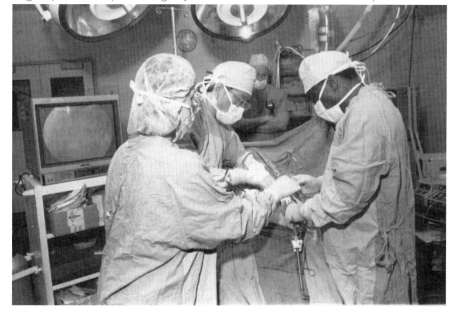
A team performing laparoscopic surgery at Windsor Western Hospital are [from left]: operating room nurse Joanne Treverton, Dr. John Yee and Dr. Akpata.

WINDSOR WESTERN LEADS IN LAPAROSCOPIC CHOLECYSTECTOMY PROCEDURES

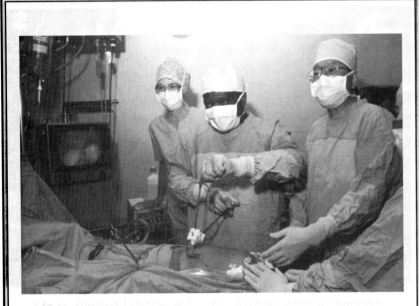

Since first introduced to the community at Windsor Western, over one hundred (100) Laparoscopic Cholecystectomy procedures have been successfully completed. Developed by the French, the procedure was first performed in Canada less than two years ago and in that short time, has revolutionized gallbladder surgery.

Dr. Michael Akpata, who has performed many of the procedures at Windsor Western, states that prior to this latest technology, major surgery for gallbladder included up to seven or more days in the hospital, five to six weeks of recovery and a long period of discomfort to the patient.

This new surgical procedure offers numerous advantages for the patient including being safer; resulting in a shorter length of stay which is usually less than two days, and provides significantly less pain and discomfort.

Surgeons, using a laparocscope, (a tube inserted through a 2 cm incision in the abdomen) can view what they are doing on a television screen. Operating through three tiny incisions, the structures are magnified up to sixteen times the size. The gallbladder is clamped off, cut and pulled out through the tube.

Dr. Akpata says he is ready to take the next step due to continuing advanced technology in laparoscopic surgery. Laparoscopic hernia procedures, bowel surgery, and hiatal hernia repairs have since begun. He is proud that Windsor Western is currently the leader in laparoscopic cholecystectomy procedures, noting that the hospital is recognized for its innovations in new and proactive approaches.

A team performing laparoscopic surgery at Windsor Western Hospital are [from left]: operating room nurse Virginia Whittal, Dr. Akpata, Dr. John Yee and Joanne Treverton. Article from the Windsor Western Hospital newsletter.

Surgical innovation eases pain of gallbladder removal

By Ellen van Wageningen
Star Medical Reporter

Having her gallbladder out was much simpler and less painful than she'd imagined, says Cathy Roberts.

She had the surgery one day and was home the next.

"I'm fully recovered and I haven't been home a week," Roberts said recently. Her gallbladder was removed Aug. 24.

The 29-year-old waitress was one of the first to have the new type of gallbladder surgery done in Windsor. In the last year many Windsorites have been going to London for the less painful surgery, said Dr. Murray Girotti, head of general surgery at Victoria Hospital.

Dr. Michael Akpata, Roberts' surgeon, said he was sold on the technique — called laparoscopic cholecystectomy — after completing the training to do it this spring.

A handful of other Windsor surgeons have taken the training and all four Windsor hospitals are in the process of ordering the equipment. Half a dozen people have had the operation in Windsor. Several Leamington surgeons are also considering adopting the technique.

"I'm intrigued by the body response to this thing," Akpata said.

In the traditional gallbladder operation the surgeon makes an incision in the abdomen and removes the diseased organ.

Using a laparoscope, a tube inserted through a 2-cm incision in the patient's navel, the surgeon can watch what he's doing on a television screen. The surgeon operates through three tiny, 0.5-cm incisions with specially designed tools. The gallbladder is clamped off, cut free and pulled up through the tube. The average gallbladder, located under the liver, is about 8 cm long.

Surgeons at Victoria Hospital have been using the technique for a year. Girotti is now teaching other surgeons to use laparoscopy, which is catching on like wildfire.

"It's probably one of the most exciting things that's happened to general surgery in the last 15 to 20 years," he said.

The biggest advantage to removing gallbladders with a laparoscope is to the patient. It's less painful and the recovery time is shorter.

At Victoria Hospital the average stay for patients who have their gallbladders removed with laparoscopy is two days. With older techniques the average stay is three to five days.

The average absence from work after the new treatment is two weeks, compared to as long as six weeks after standard surgery.

IN THE LAST year all but 20 of the 350 patients who had gallbladder surgery at Victoria Hospital chose the new procedure.

Not everyone is a candidate. Pregnant women are disqualified because of the danger to their babies. Heart conditions, previous strokes and previous operations all make laparoscopic surgery more risky.

Dr. George Stojanovic, head of general surgery at Windsor Western Hospital, was skeptical when he heard about laparoscopic cholecystectomy.

"I thought it was somehow a sort of trend that was going to pass," he said. "When I realized I was wrong I went and took the course."

Akpata and Stojanovic estimate that about 800 Windsor and Essex County residents have their gallbladders removed every year.

Demand for the new surgery is patient-driven, Stojanovic says. Why would anyone stay in hospital for five days if they could be out in two? Spend a month recovering when it could take only a week or two?

The equipment to perform laparoscopy costs between $40,000 and $60,000. Surgeons use $500 worth of disposable equipment for each operation, compared to $100 for the standard operation.

The laparoscopic surgery takes 15 to 30 minutes longer, but times are dropping as surgeons become more proficient, Akpata said.

The most experienced surgeons in Canada are starting to use laparoscopy to remove cancerous pieces of the bowel, kidney and lung. Gynecologists are using laparoscopic surgery to remove ovarian cysts and sterilize women. Orthopedic surgeons use a similar technique to remove and repair knee ligaments.

Discussions about laparoscopic surgery are expected to take up two days of the annual meeting of Canadian Royal College of Physicians and Surgeons in September.

Girotti and Akpata say they believe it's the wave of the future in surgery.

Dr. Michael Akpata was featured in an article after removing the gallbladder of a 29-year-old waitress. The Windsor Star, September 5, 1991.

procedure would become state of the art for surgery in the future.

The next step was to be precepted by a laparoscopic specialist for the first two cases prior to doing cases on my own. I arranged for Dr. Murray Girotti, who was my course coordinator at Victoria Hospital to come to Windsor to precept my first case at Windsor Western. The Chief of Surgery was also included for his first case on that same day.

The supervisor of the operating room was willing to pay extra staff on a Saturday so it could be carried out in a quiet atmosphere away from the usual daily activity of the operating room.

My first patient was a lady in her seventies who owned and ran an insurance business. She was a golfer, medically fit and anxious to undergo this new procedure. Prior to surgery, I explained the procedure and possible complications. She signed my informed consent, a copy of which was given to her to take home for additional reading.

On August 10, 1991, I was proud to have carried out my first precepted laparoscopic cholecystectomy case in Windsor at Windsor Western and appreciated the help of Dr. Girotti. That evening I was so anxious that I called the hospital several times to see how my patient was doing. The following day, after my regular church service, I quickly went to the hospital to see her even though I was confident that everything had gone well during the surgery.

When I arrived at the hospital, this seventy year old lady shocked and surprised me. There she was sitting in a chair in the hallway outside of her room reading a newspaper. When I asked her how she felt, she replied that she was feeling very well, wanted to go home and asked when she could return to playing golf.

I was quite pleased with this result.

After checking the incisions, I discharged her home for the following day with instructions to see me in one week at the office.

My second patient was a waitress and underwent her procedure on August 24, 1991 again under the preceptorship of Dr. Girotti. When I saw her the next day, she also looked well and was anxious to be discharged.

This was further proof to me as to the advantages of this procedure and that laparoscopy would definitely be the way of the future.

Now that I had done my first two required cases, I was given privileges at Windsor Western to continue to perform laparoscopic cholecystectomy there. I applied for privileges and was approved at Hôtel Dieu and Grace Hospitals. Word spread quickly in the community and patients began requesting laparoscopy or 'this new keyhole surgery' as they called it.

My surgical practice mushroomed as I was one of the first to perform this procedure and within a year I had done approximately 150 cases.

I was fortunate enough to have had Dr. John Yee, a general practitioner and a very good friend of mine who was willing to assist me from the beginning. He had already been assisting on many of my other surgeries and took a special interest in laparoscopy.

An important aspect of laparoscopy is having an excellent assistant with a steady hand who can direct the camera properly. This was one of his greater abilities and I am forever indebted to him for his many years of help. As time went on, I decided to take more in-depth courses to advance in laparoscopic procedures and be able to do more of my abdominal cases laparoscopically.

Laparoscopic surgery was certainly not without the possibility of complications regardless of the many advantages. It was a new frontier and several articles had been written about the myriad of serious problems resulting from surgery done by inexperienced physicians.

There was not even an agreeable consensus among the surgeons in Windsor as to whether this type of surgery would continue as predicted or become a passing fad.

On one occasion, Dr. Charles Pearce, Chief of Surgery at Hôtel Dieu, approached me to help draft the credentialing regulations for these procedures. At that time, I was the most experienced in the field for laparoscopic cholecystectomy. I wrote to the hospitals where I had undertaken my courses to get input for their credentialing system.

Once the regulations were put together and handed over to the Chief of Surgery, it became the requirement for any surgeon to fulfill before being granted privileges. Briefly, the guidelines for credentialing were as follows:

• Only general surgeons experienced in open cholecystectomy and the management of potential complications should perform laparoscopic cholecystectomy.

• The physician should attend an approved training course, usually two days in length, during which time the individual is exposed to lectures entailing the basics in laparoscopy, its complications and including an animal lab. The training program should also include observation of surgery on humans in the operating room.

• Upon arrival back in Windsor, the surgeon must perform at least two cases on his own, under the supervision of an experienced laparoscopist. Satisfactory performance by the surgeon should be in writing by the preceptor before proceeding on his own.

Several of my colleagues approached me to precept them during their first two cases. At other times, I was called to help with unusual situations. I was proud to see many of my colleagues interested in learning this new procedure which was becoming state of the art.

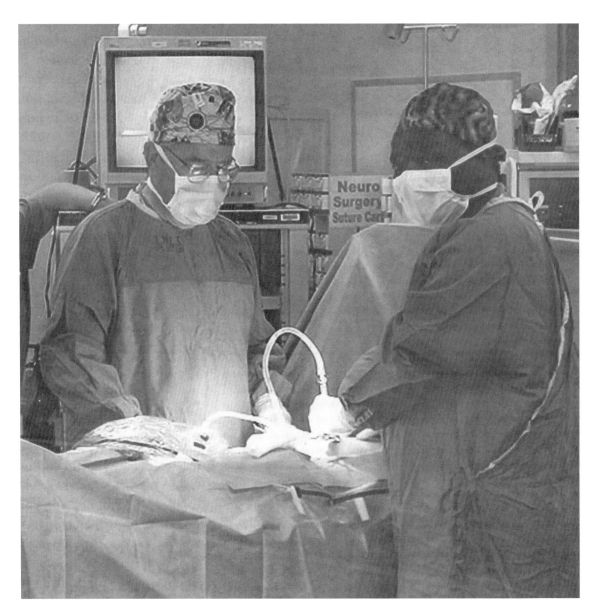
Dr. Akpata assisted by Dr. Charles Pearce performing surgery.

CHAPTER TWENTY ONE
TRAINING IN ADVANCED LAPAROSCOPY

Advanced laparoscopy requires a lot of training as it is quite complex. I decided to undertake several courses before plunging into this next stage of minimally invasive surgery. The first course I attended was held at Norwalk, Connecticut, February 6-7, 1992 under the auspices of the Auto Suture Company.

I was quite pleased to receive an invitation to attend this conference of hands-on surgery. The two day course was very elaborate, including the learning of laparoscopic intra-abdominal suturing and surgical procedures of the upper and lower gastrointestinal tract carried out in an animal lab.

In spite of my many years of doing surgery, nothing could have prepared me for the difficulty of 'blind suturing'. We were given a box covered in clear plastic through which long handled instruments were inserted to practice the suturing technique with the image portrayed on a screen in front of us.

I spent many nights after that course sitting in my office at home working to perfect this art form. I dare say, the young surgeons today have the advantage of growing up playing video games which certainly helps with the manual dexterity needed for this procedure.

The course instructors were very experienced and very patient. Following the two-day course, I felt energized to continue my training in advanced laparoscopic surgery as I could definitely see the benefits to it.

In April 1992, I again decided to spend some further time at the Saskatoon City Hospital under the directorship of Dr. Demetrius Litwin. As before, I had to be registered with the College of Physicians and Surgeons of Saskatchewan and obtain approval from the Director of Continuing Medical Education at the hospital. I had hands-on training for a week and either assisted or performed practically every procedure that could be done laparoscopically at that time.

I was also on call in the evenings if any case came in through the emergency room such as acute appendicitis. This was time well spent as it helped immensely with my dexterity and overall experience.

In June of 1992, I attended another two-day course in advanced laparoscopic surgery in Vancouver, sponsored by the Auto Suture Company. I cannot thank this company enough for all the assistance in making sure that several of us throughout the country were exposed to the various types of procedures available.

The more procedures we learned, the more specific instruments would be introduced and sold to the hospitals, the company this time being the beneficiary.

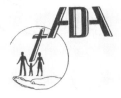

Letter granting privileges to Dr. Michael Akpata in advanced laparoscopic surgery by Frank N. Bagatto.

Coming back home to Windsor, I started doing advanced laparoscopic procedures in earnest. This required the training of the operating room nurses, since no other general surgeon was interested at least at that time in doing advanced laparoscopic procedures.

Most of my work was being done at Windsor Western as the administration was very keen on being at the forefront of any new surgical advances.

The day prior to any new procedure, I went over each step of the surgery along with the instrumentation needed with the two nurses scheduled to be with me the following day. That evening they would meet at my home along with my assistant, Dr. John Yee, to watch a teaching video of that procedure.

I realized that a successful surgical outcome depended on all staff members being knowledgeable and able to work together as a team.

As well, a technician from the Auto Suture Company was always on hand during the case to guide the nurses.

My first advanced case was called Nissen fundoplication, a procedure used to treat hiatus hernia with reflux which has not responded well to medical therapy. It involves wrapping the upper part of the stomach around the lower part of the esophagus to prevent food contents in the stomach from reversing and entering the esophagus or trachea (windpipe).

Some of the available nursing staff and a few of my colleagues came in to watch the procedure at different times as it was the first one being done in the city. Everything went well and the patient was fit to be discharged home in two days as compared to the previous seven to ten days with the open method. I was pleased and encouraged with these results.

In these early days, patients were carefully chosen as there was quite a learning curve involved to this technique. Only those with no other health issues such as high blood pressure, diabetes and heart problems were offered the choice. Also they must not have had any previous abdominal surgery with resulting adhesions.

Following gastroscopy showing the presence of acid reflux from the stomach, the patients were chosen based on their performance in specific tests which measured the pressure at the gastroesophageal junction and the amount of acid entering the esophagus. These tests were done in London and would ultimately indicate the need for this laparoscopic procedure.

The next advanced procedure I did was the resection and removal of a portion of the large bowel on the right side for cancer in a middle-aged lady. I was still encouraged with laparoscopy resulting in less pain and shorter hospital stays.

Soon after, I did my first operation on the stomach laparoscopically which was called posterior vagotomy and seromyotomy. This is done for the treatment of chronic duodenal ulcer that has been unresponsive to medical therapy thus helping to reduce the amount of acid produced in the stomach.

At this point, I was approached by the chief of surgery at Windsor Western about the idea of getting more reusable equipment as most of the instruments I was using were disposable and more costly. I was allowed to do eight more cases of laparoscopic surgery with the disposable equipment and then report to the chief of surgery in order to reassess the costs in relation to the overall operating room budget.

Lloyd Preston, Chief Executive Officer of the hospital, was well known to run a very tight ship. He also was concerned about whether the higher operating cost of these new procedures would balance the shorter length of hospital stay. I was soon called into his office for a discussion.

He informed me that the program had been well received by him, the chief of surgery and the hospital as a whole and to some extent by the general surgeons. He suggested that I do an impact study regarding the cost of the new laparoscopic procedures versus the open standard method and compare the advantages of both methods especially in regards to the response of the patients. We made arrangements to get together at a later date to share this information.

Everyone in the hospital including the director of the operating room, the staff and the CEO himself were pleased to know that Windsor Western was in the forefront in advanced laparoscopic procedures.

This request from the CEO was a tall order for me to fulfill. Of course as a surgeon, my overall interest was to continue with my advanced laparoscopic procedures and not have to worry about any financial aspect. On the other hand I realized that for the hospital to function properly there had to be a balanced budget.

I was a bit concerned about the outcome of this impact study. The easiest part of the procedure was to identify the cost of the old methods which was obtained through hospital statistical records. I was able to work with the director of the operating room, the purchasing agent as well as the Auto Suture Company, to put together all the equipment costs. We also looked at purchasing more reusable instruments rather than the disposable ones the company had supplied us in the beginning. Once I was able to put together what I felt to be an honest and fair assessment, I approached the CEO.

To my surprise, he had done a separate study of his own. He was a very competent manager and I was about to see the side of him known for keeping the hospital books financially balanced.

As I presented information from my itemized list, he sat in front of me turning pages of his own, nodding in agreement and sometimes giving me facts before I had a chance to present them. This was a man who always did his homework. At the end of our discussion, he agreed that I should proceed with laparoscopic procedures in the hospital to the extent that I was already trained to do.

The reason for his decision was because the financial requirements were not as exorbitant as he had thought previously. Secondly, he was aware of the shorter hospital stay of laparoscopic patients as compared to the open method.

One important aspect that came out of this study involved the use of disposable equipment. I was advised that I had to keep disposable items to a minimum and therefore the hospital would purchase as many reusable instruments as possible for me to be able to continue with my work.

CHAPTER TWENTY TWO
SYMPOSIUM ON MINIMAL ACCESS SURGERY

The first International Symposium on Minimal Access Surgery was held at the Saskatoon City Hospital under the directorship of Dr. Demetrius Litwin on August 7-8, 1992. It covered a broad spectrum of laparoscopic surgery including removal of the gallbladder, management of its complications and exploration of the bile ducts.

I shall not attempt to enumerate all the topics that were discussed but for simplicity they included practically anything that could be done surgically in the abdomen

PHOTO GALLERY

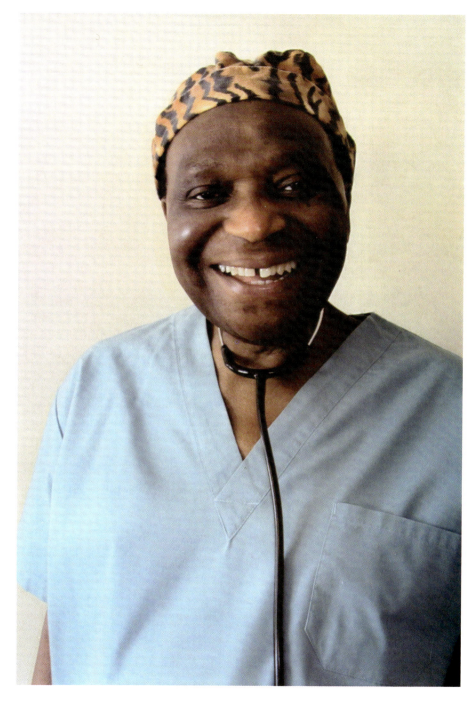

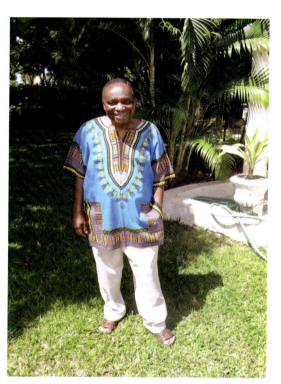

[above] Dr. Akpata at home in Barbados.

[left] Dr. Michael Akpata in his scrubs.

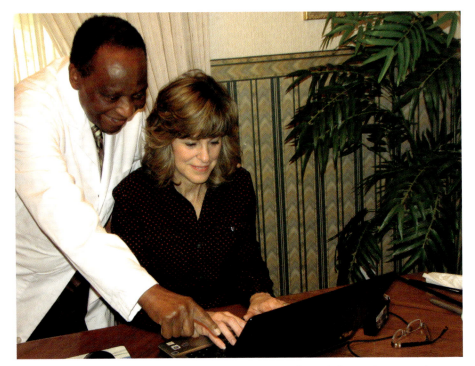

Dr. Michael Akpata with his secretary, Carol Attenborough

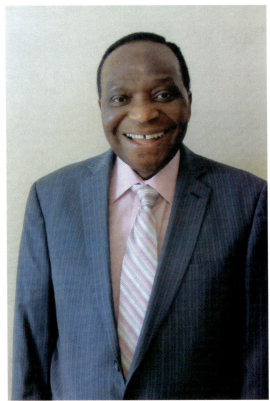

[above] Dr. Akpata in his regular outfit.

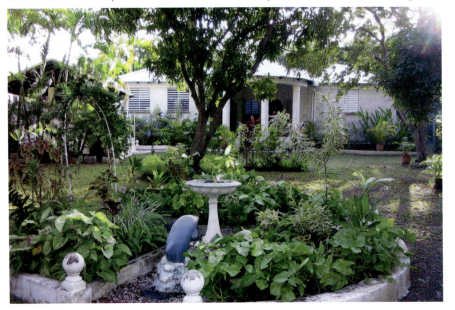

[left] Dr. Akpata's home in Barbados.

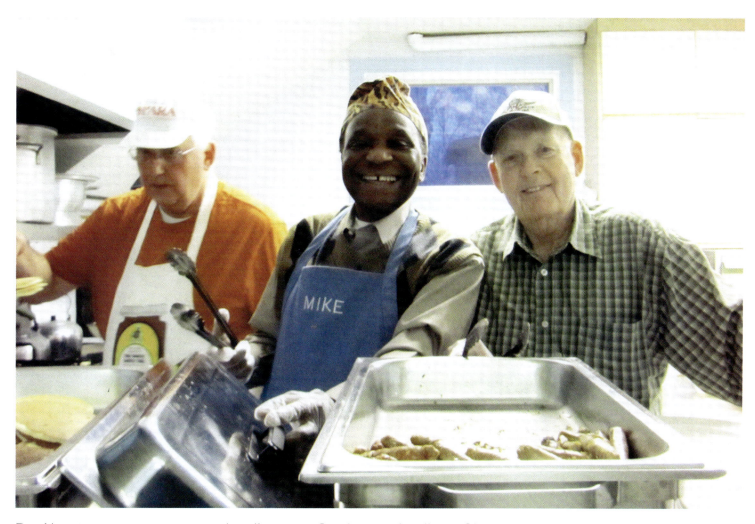

Dr. Akpata serves at a pancake dinner at St. James Anglican Church with [left] Rod Reid and Les Branch.

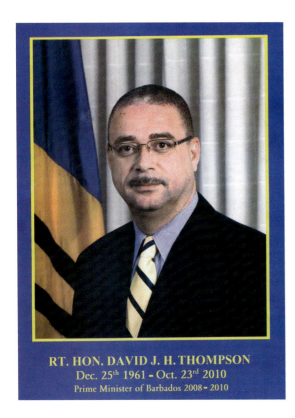

[above] Rt. Hon. David J. H. Thompson, Prime Minister of Barbados 2008-2010 (deceased).

[right] A Report To Our Community Hotel-Dieu Grace Hospital newsletter group photo, April 2001-2002.

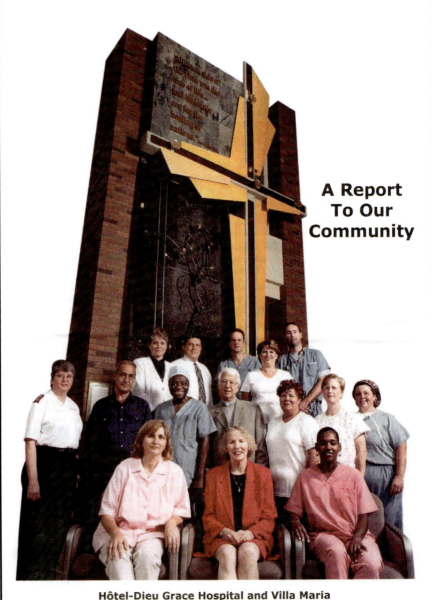

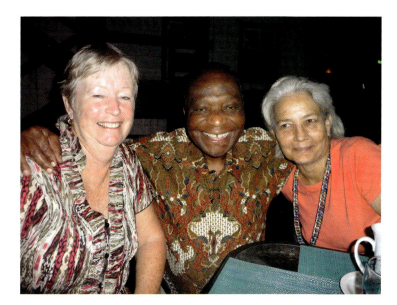

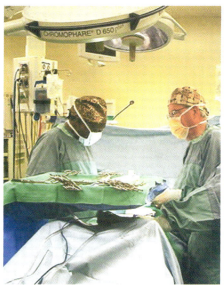

(left) Dr. Akpata with Dr. Charles Pearce performing surgery.

[above] Dr. Akpata with Lynda Lewis [left], assistant administrator and Sian Monteith, operating room supervisor of Bayview Hospital, Barbados.

[right] Dr. Michael Akpata writing his book.

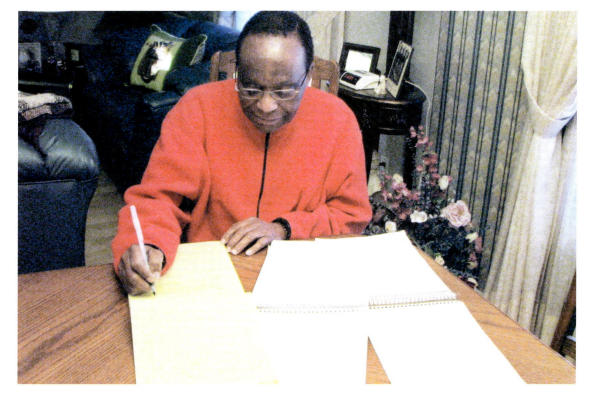

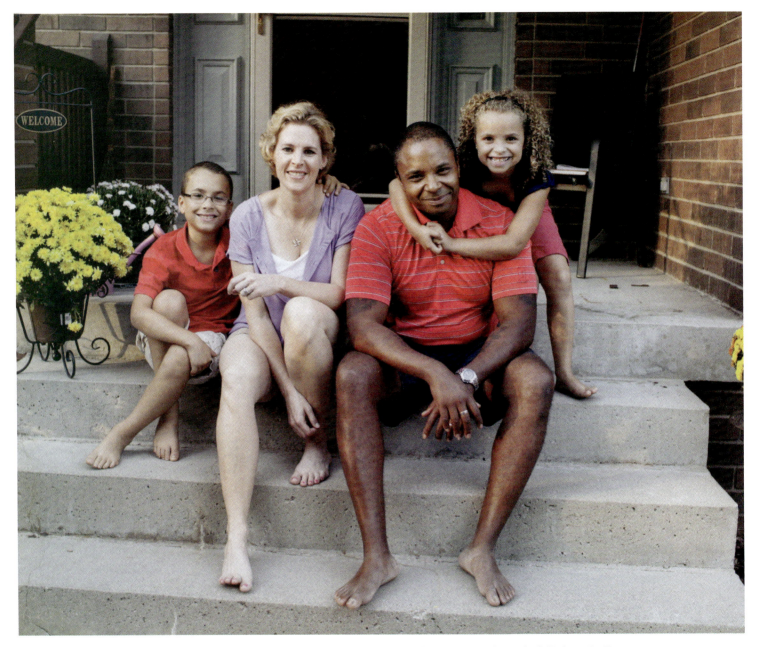

Dr. Akpata's eldest son Michael with his family [from left]: Reece, Sheri, Michael, Regan.

Dr. Akpata's daughter Michelle with her family [from left]: Shawn, Ayla, Michelle, Evan.

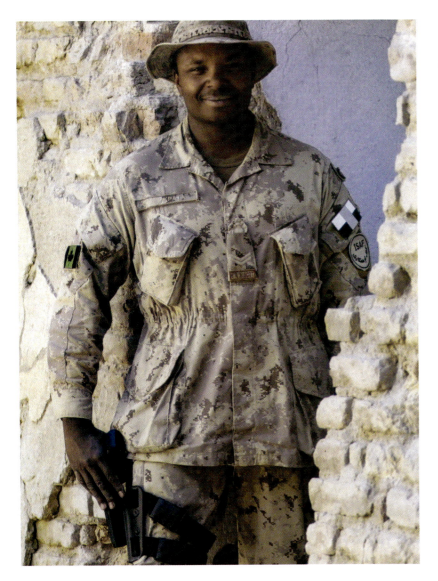

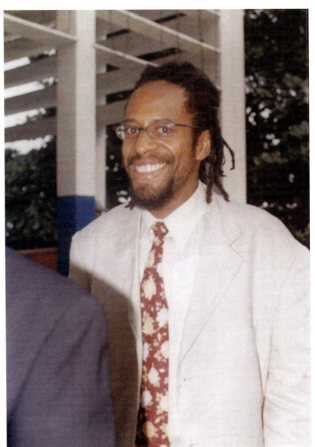

[left] Dr. Akpata's son Michael who voluntarily served in Afganistan with the Canadian Armed Forces. Also a Windsor police officer.

[right] Dr. Akpata's youngest son John, a poet and musician.

and pelvis including routine cases like appendectomy (removal of the appendix) and hernia repair.

These were the pioneering days of laparoscopy and certain names stood out as world renowned experts. Several of them were at this meeting including Dr. Philippe Mouret, the French surgeon who was the first to perform the removal of a diseased gallbladder laparoscopically in Leon, France in 1987. Also present were Dr. Michel Gagner, Dr. Lawrence Way, Dr. Namir Katkhouda and Dr. Karl Zucker. There were other professors of laparoscopic surgery who were well known to me such as Dr. Murray Girotti and Dr. Demetrius Litwin because of their roles in my own personal training.

One could see that the speakers came from a cross-section of veritable laparoscopic surgeons from the United States, Canada and France. The discussions were very well handled by the respective speakers and very informative.

Prior to leaving Windsor for the symposium, I had spoken to the management of both Windsor Western and Hôtel Dieu requesting that at least two nurses from each institution be allowed to accompany me to this symposium. I knew it was vital that the nursing staff be educated in advanced laparoscopy and have an opportunity to speak with the sales representatives regarding the purchase and care of instruments.

During this symposium, there were several items donated by the various companies as door prizes including a set of very expensive golf clubs. I was out in the hallway attending the many equipment booths with the nurses from our two Windsor hospitals when I heard my name paged.

To my surprise, I was the lucky winner of these golf clubs. Ironic for someone who does not golf. Many knew their value and offered to buy them. I thanked them for their offers but had decided to take them home to my son who was an avid golfer.

Maybe there was a message here that it was time for me to slow down and 'smell the roses'.

CHAPTER TWENTY THREE
SOCIETY FOR LAPAROSCOPIC AND ENDOSCOPIC SURGERY

The Canadian Society for Laparoscopic and Endoscopic Surgery is a non-profit organization and a registered national society recognized by the Royal College of Physicians and Surgeons of Canada. The objectives of the society are to provide leadership in both endoscopic and laparoscopic surgery and stimulate research and teaching in both of these aspects. It also provides a forum for the members to present papers at organized meetings. It therefore serves as a way to keep members updated with the lat-

THE SOCIETY OF LAPAROENDOSCOPIC SURGEONS

Michael Akpata, MD

has been elected
to membership in
the Society of Laparoendoscopic Surgeons

Joseph A. Gurri, MD
Membership Chairman

Paul A. Wetter, MD
Chairman, Board of Trustees

Dr. Michael Akpata's certificate of membership to the Society of Laparoendoscopic Surgeons.

est innovations in minimally invasive surgery and endoscopy.

Membership includes gynecologists, general surgeons, urologists and other health professionals in Canada, the U.S. and abroad.

Since I had taken so many courses in laparoscopic surgery and endoscopy, I felt it would be in my best interest to join the society. The prerequisites to become a member include the following:

• Completed and signed application form.
• Copy of certificate of one's specialty plus MD and any others.
• Two copies of a letter of recommendation from the instructor.
• Two copies of a letter of recommendation from the current Chief of Surgery.

I obtained a letter of recommendation from Dr. Murray Girotti who was my first instructor in laparoscopic cholecystectomy and from Dr. Charles Pearce, Chief of Surgery at Hôtel Dieu. Once I fulfilled the above requirements, I was accepted into this important society.

CHAPTER TWENTY FOUR
POST GRADUATE COURSE - ADVANCED LAPAROSCOPY

I attended a post graduate course in Charleston, South Carolina with the main emphasis on advanced laparoscopic procedures from April 1-4, 1993. Several experts

Dr. Michael Akpata's letter of recommendation from Dr. Charles Pearce.

were invited to participate in the program. The topics discussed included many diverse advanced procedures and their possible complications. It was informative to hear other surgeons present discuss their experiences in these advanced procedures.

At one stage during the conference, the moderator wanted to find out how many of the surgeons present were already trained in minimally invasive surgery. He started by asking for a show of hands from members who were performing laparoscopic cholecystectomy and practically every surgeon in the hall put up his hand.

As he went through the list of the many laparoscopic procedures being done at that time, the number of members raising their hands gradually dropped. Of the 500 who were asked how many had done laparoscopic splenectomy (removal of the spleen), only three hands went up, including mine.

He congratulated the three of us and encouraged everyone present to press on with the learning process of advanced laparoscopy as it was destined to be the future method of surgery.

During that evening, we had a dinner cruise around the harbor area on the 'Spirit of Charleston'. I was approached by one of my fellow surgeons who began to quiz me about all these procedures the moderator had discussed earlier that morning.

"Correct me if I am wrong, but I saw your hand up in response to each of the procedures he asked about. You must be an excellent and aggressive surgeon to have learned and had the opportunity to perform all those procedures within two years!"

I thanked him for his compliments and explained I had attended many courses involving hands-on procedures across Canada and the U.S. and I planned to continue in order to be more proficient.

At that point, he beckoned to his wife who was close by to come and join us. He proceeded to say to his wife, "Honey, this is the man I told you about earlier who has had a lot of laparoscopic experience."

Then he turned to me and said, "You must be very rich with a yacht, a mansion and a fancy car, right?"

At this point, I burst out laughing. "Sir, you forget that we are from Canada and the health care system is controlled by each province whereby procedures are coded and payment is standardized."

He replied, "I am sure you still make more money than I do. OK, what do you get for doing an inguinal hernia repair?" I replied that I would be paid in the range of $250 for this procedure regardless of which method I used. There was no additional charge for doing a case laparoscopically and this fee included any follow up care.

"What, you have to be joking! There is no way I would even get out of bed for that amount of money even if they tied a rope around my neck and dragged me to the operating table," the American surgeon replied.

"Now you know why I have no yacht or expensive house. For every dollar that I make, 39 cents goes to running my office and the remaining 61 cents is taxed at the rate of 50% by our government. The balance is mine to spend to take care of my household and car expenses, life insurance and retirement savings."

We shook hands and parted company while he walked away shaking his head.

The next meeting of the Society of Laparoscopy and Endoscopy that I attended was the fourth annual conference at the Hyatt Regency Grand Cypress, Orlando, Florida from December 7-9, 1995. Again my objective was to be at the forefront of laparoscopic surgery. This was a worthwhile conference, for it energized and reinforced in me the need for these new procedures. It also gave me the confidence that I was keeping up to date with the latest developments.

Following this course, there was another seminar in Montreal in 1997 sponsored by the Auto Suture Company. This was a more specific course involving a full day workshop in laparoscopic inguinal hernia repair and another day in Nissen Fundoplication.

These hands-on workshops were extremely helpful in increasing my manual dexterity to perform these procedures.

My referral practice was growing by leaps and bounds. Family physicians were aware of my intense dedication to the practice of advanced laparoscopic surgery. Laparoscopy was basically a patient-driven surgery as the public became more aware of its advantages.

When I first arrived in Windsor in 1980, a 44-year-old lady with chronic ulcerative colitis that was being treated medically, was referred to me. She had a follow-up colonoscopy on an annual basis and the disease was kept under control using the specific medicines prescribed for her.

After several years of this treatment, she developed complications including recurrent rectal bleeding, severe weight loss and chronic abdominal pain. She was no longer responding to treatment medically and there was a concern for possible development of colon cancer. A colonoscopy revealed severe diffuse ulcerative colitis (inflammation of the bowel with open sores or ulcers) and biopsy of the mucosa (lining of the bowel) showed evidence of dysplasia. She was now one step closer to developing bowel cancer.

Her condition became much worse and I therefore suggested that she should have a total colectomy with possible ileostomy. This would involve removal of the entire large bowel and rectum with the formation of a permanent opening on the abdominal wall which would require wearing a pouch to collect the waste products.

This lady absolutely refused to have this surgery done.

I decided to send her to a gastroenterologist in London, Ontario for assessment and follow-up colonoscopy. The gastroenterologist agreed with me that this patient required surgery as soon as possible to alleviate her symptoms and prevent an even worse situation from happening.

He referred her to a well-respected and competent general surgeon at Victoria Hospital in London. She was again advised that at this point, surgery was the only option left to her. She was given a date for laparoscopic colectomy with endo-anal pull-through hopefully preventing an ileostomy. She reluctantly agreed to go ahead with this surgery.

I saw her several times in my office encouraging her, praising the surgical team in London and again stressing that this was still her best option.

On the assigned date for surgery, as she was being wheeled into the waiting area outside the operating room at Victoria Hospital, she asked if I was going to be there to do the surgery.

When she was told that the surgeon she had been seeing in London would be the one to do the surgery, she yelled, "Stop. Let me out of this bed. I want to go back home to Windsor. I thought Dr Akpata was going to be here to do my surgery."

She was quite adamant in her decision. Both the gastroenterologist and the surgeon had a very intensive discussion with this patient but she would not change her mind. On this basis she was discharged back home to Windsor without surgery.

Before she arrived home, I received an urgent telephone call from the surgeon to inform me of the problem that had arisen. He related the day's events to me and we had an in-depth discussion on what the next step should be.

Shortly after, I received a telephone call from the patient herself who wanted to see me right away in my office. She told me what had happened and as much as I was upset with her, I did not lose my temper. I knew she was under tremendous stress and did not want to have a permanent ileostomy.

I reminded her that we had had a long discussion about this surgery including the possible complications, the high risk of her developing cancer of the colon or rectum and we were not set up in Windsor yet to handle this case laparoscopically.

She apologized for cancelling the surgery and that is when I told her that she should have notified the surgeon long before the date of the planned surgery as the time set aside in the operating room for her was wasted. She was advised to stay on her medications.

I was surprised to receive a call from Dr. Murray Girotti offering me one day of surgical privileges at Victoria Hospital, to perform this procedure under his supervision. I was delighted because hospitals do not generally give one day privileges. I accepted his generous offer.

I then called the patient into my office and explained what had transpired and impressed upon her the most unusual circumstance which had just happened. I am sure this would never have happened except for my close relationship with Dr. Girotti during the many past months of laparoscopic work.

On February 3, 1994, I performed a laparoscopic endo-anal pull-through procedure on my patient, assisted by the chief surgical resident and with Dr. Girotti in attendance. She did very well and did not require an ileostomy. She has a colonoscopy on an annual basis to make sure there are no recurring signs of cancer.

My experience with Dr. Girotti will never be forgotten. This very good friend, outstanding surgeon and educator recently passed away due to ill health. I will never forget him.

CHAPTER TWENTY FIVE
CBC TELEVISION INTERVIEWS

My first interview with the Canadian Broadcasting Corporation in Windsor was in 1988. There was an interest in a procedure called pancreaticoduodenectomy or Whipple's, for carcinoma of the head of the pancreas which I had been doing since coming to the city. There was one other surgeon also trained in this procedure who arrived a few months before me. Until that time, patients from Windsor and vicinity with pancreatic cancer were required to go either to London, Toronto or Detroit for surgery. Needless to say, I was quite humbled and pleased to undergo this interview.

The moderator first asked me questions about my training in this aspect of surgical practice. I told him I had been fortunate to be taught by the professor of hepatobiliary and pancreatic surgery who took special interest in me during my residency at the University of Alberta.

The interviewer had a list of questions, including what symptoms the patient presented to his family doctor, my investigation and management and the outcome of my surgical procedures.

Usually only the diseased portion of the pancreas is removed but due to its proximity to the stomach and other organs, it requires a lot of dissecting and removal of other parts to have a successful outcome. This can take anywhere up to eight hours to do and requires a dedicated team. The postoperative care is extremely important and can be very complex.

Most of my patients had a reasonable outcome. This interview lasted about an hour and I thanked the interviewer for the opportunity to be on the show to discuss this disease.

In 1993, I again received a request for a television interview regarding the new and innovative laparoscopy procedures which were then being performed in Windsor. I was accompanied by Dr. David Wonham, Chief of Surgery at Windsor Western.

There was a discussion about the history of laparoscopy and its application in all aspects of general surgery. Excerpts of some videos of the procedures I had performed were shown. By this time, I had done many laparoscopic cholecystectomy cases. But, I also had been involved in numerous advanced laparoscopic cases, most of them new to Windsor. We had a good question and answer period and I was quite pleased with the result.

At the end of the interview, we were both complimented for our dedication and interest in being at the forefront of the development of laparoscopy in Windsor.

CHAPTER TWENTY SIX
CARIBBEAN CONNECTION

My first trip to the Caribbean was by chance and a lucky draw. During one of my office days, the mail carrier brought a registered letter addressed to me. As registered mail sometimes brings bad news, I opened and read the contents with some trepidation. Imagine my surprise when I read that I had won a trip for two to Aruba, courtesy of Esso Canada. I discussed this with my secretary, who felt as I did, that it was just another hoax.

Unknown to me, there had been a random draw for the purpose of advertisement for clients who held Esso gas credit cards. It stated that my card number had randomly been chosen in the draw for a free trip.

Esso Canada verified my name, address and card number and informed me the prize was a trip for two people to Aruba, all expenses paid. Once I notified the trip's travel agent, the flight and hotels in Toronto and Aruba were booked. I was grateful and amazed that I had actually won the draw. This trip was my first introduction to a Caribbean island and certainly would not be my last.

The following year, I went on a Caribbean cruise which included the port of Barbados, a very beautiful island and probably the best of all the islands visited during that cruise. The island itself was very clean, the food was great and all the amenities we have in Canada were available. More important, the residents of the island were religious, polite and friendly.

Although we were only in Barbados for one day, we were able to contact Dr. Jerry Emtage, a good friend who had worked in Windsor with us. He is an Urologist who had practiced at Windsor Western for several years prior to moving back to his home in Barbados. We had lunch at the 'Waterfront Café' where he told us about Bayview Hospital, a private institution and his main place of practice. He first introduced us to the hospital executive director, the chief of surgery and the entire operating room staff before a guided tour of the hospital.

Jerry sang my praises about laparoscopy and said that I had the most experience of anyone he knew.

Mr. Arthur Edghill, Chief of Surgery, remarked that several of their surgeons were interested in learning laparoscopic cholecystectomy and wondered if it would be possible to set up a program for them to attend either in Canada or in Barbados. He suggested that if I was interested, I could possibly return at a later date to work out the logistics.

The consensus was that it would be easier for me to teach in Barbados rather than all of them coming to Canada. This would have included applying for temporary registration with the College of Physicians and Surgeons in Ontario in addition to the cost of flight, lodging and registration fees.

I made arrangements to return to Barbados in the summer of 1993 to begin a teaching program. I was required to send him my credentials so that he could register me with the Medical Board of Barbados and also request hospital privileges for me to teach there.

Once all the paperwork had been carried out, I returned to Barbados on January 17, 1994 with an experienced technician from the Auto Suture Company and with all the necessary equipment for setting up the program. His company was very gracious to supply the instruments needed, free of charge, for this course with the stipulation that any materials not used would be available for purchase by the hospital at a nominal fee.

I was provided with a letter of introduction for us to present to the Customs and Immigration staff to allow us to bring in the equipment. Upon our arrival at the airport in Barbados, we were met by Lynda Lewis, Assistant Hospital Administrator, and Sian Monteith, Operating Theatre Supervisor, who took us to our place of lodging which was a beautiful villa called 'Tantalus'. It was on the beach of the west coast and owned by a couple who also had a tourist party boat called the 'Jolly Roger'.

On January 18, 1994, after becoming acquainted with one another, we started our formal course in laparoscopic cholecystectomy. The course involved the introduction of the equipment including the television monitor, the carbon dioxide machine and the hand instruments. The technician described the use and function of each instrument. I then showed a narrated video of the procedure and discussed the following topics:

• The history of laparoscopic cholecystectomy.
• Complications and contraindications.
• Precautionary measures.

The second day involved an animal workshop. This procedure was carried out at a local veterinary clinic using pigs that were already compromised medically.

I showed each surgeon the basics, including the insertion of the needle in order

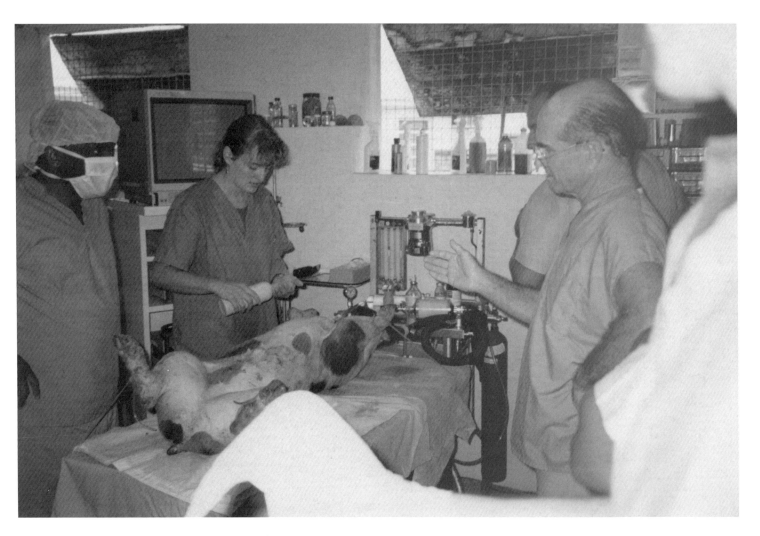

Dr. Akpata [left] instructing Mr. Arthur Edghill, General Surgeon and Chairman of the Board of Directors at Bayview Hospital, and other surgeons preparing for an animal workshop at a veterinary clinic in Barbados.

to inflate the abdomen with carbon dioxide, how to insert the ports and the actual dissection of the gallbladder with its removal from the abdomen.

The participants each had an opportunity to be involved with the hands-on aspect with guidance from myself and the technician. Just as we had done in Canada, the participants took turns being the operating surgeon, camera man and assistant.

On days 3, 4 and 5, we had the opportunity to operate on patients who had been waiting for their surgery and were willing and anxious to be part of the program. On day three, I carried out the procedure myself while one of the other surgeons acted as my assistant and another as the cameraman. On each subsequent day, the actual procedure was done by the surgeons themselves. All the cases went well without any complications.

Just as the surgeons were being taught their maneuvers, the nurses were being guided by my nurse and the Auto Suture technician showing which instrument would be needed next. Another important aspect for them was the care and handling of the instruments both during and after surgery. At the end of the sixth day, all the participants received a certificate of competence to continue on their own. The local news media was present for interviews and follow up articles in the two newspapers.

At the end of the one-week course, we were all very happy and satisfied with the

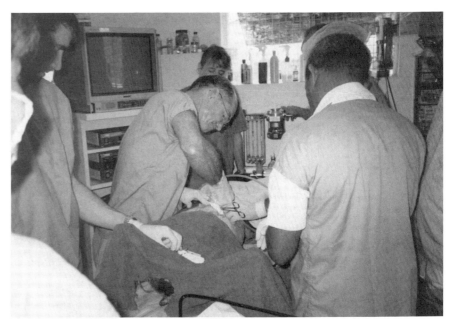
Mr. Arthur Edghill begins workshop surgery.

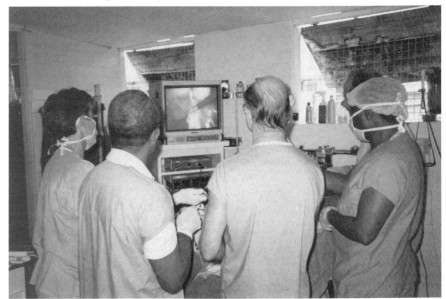
Observing surgery on a monitor.

outcome of the training and the surgeons' enthusiasm. They all agreed in the end that they did the right thing by bringing a team to Barbados to teach rather than all of them travelling to Canada. I was grateful to have had this opportunity to be of help to them.

My team spent the last few days on the island having a good time and enjoying the great weather before returning home to Canada. After a phone call to the technician's supervisor, the instruments that were not used were donated to Bayview Hospital to help them get off the ground with their laparoscopic program. This would encourage them to purchase future equipment from their company's subsidiary in Miami, Florida.

As a token for my help, I was registered as a member of the surgical staff of Bayview Hospital, since I was already registered with the Medical Board of Barbados. To maintain this position, I would be required to pay my annual dues to the hospital for continuation of my membership and also annually renew my registration with the Medical Board.

It was easy to fall in love with this island and its people. The flowers and sunshine reminded me of my home country.

The father of one of the nurses in the operating room at Bayview was a real estate agent and she kept coaxing me the entire time we were working that I should think about buying a property on the island. This was the farthest thing from my mind when I originally agreed to go for the teaching program.

To appease her, I finally said that I could spend one afternoon looking around. After seeing some extremely expensive properties, we stopped at a villa on the west coast which was vacant. Much to my surprise I found myself saying, "Yes, this is it. I will take it."

This was a huge decision and opened up a whole new dimension in my life. I would have a vacation home which could be rented out when I was in Canada and I had privileges in the private hospital where I could work, if I wanted to, whenever visiting the island.

On another occasion, the chief of surgery made arrangements for me to cover his practice while he was away on an extended holiday. This was a great experience to get to know the people of the island, the drugs available to them and to learn the functioning of their medical system.

Barbados operates under a two tier system. Everyone can attend the Queen Elizabeth Hospital which is the government institution but often must wait a lengthy time for an operation. Others who have medical insurance coverage can attend Bayview which is a private hospital. Those covered by private insurance could also travel to Florida for tests or procedures not available on the island.

Each parish or township has its own Polyclinic much like our walk-in clinics

24A JANUARY 23, 1994. Sunday Sun

HEALTH

Surgery made simpler

New technique makes it easier to operate on the gall-bladder

BARBADIAN surgeons now know more about a technique for removing gall-bladders that could greatly simplify operations.

Last week they attended a seminar which was the result of a coordinated effort among the island's medical and administrative health professionals.

The technique, called laparoscopic cholecystectomy is said to offer health, financial and cosmetic advantages over the standard operation.

Instead of cutting open the abdomen to reach the gall-bladder, as is currently the standard procedure, surgeons can simply cut several small holes in the abdomen through which they insert a camera and surgical instruments.

Though the techniques of laparoscopic cholecystectomy vary among surgeons, the procedure is usually performed by a team of three surgeons. They all look at the video monitor to watch the instruments being manoeuvered through the holes in the abdomen.

The operator manipulates long hooks, scissors and other instruments to dissect the tissue around the gall-bladder.

As this technique requires only tiny incisions, recovery is speedier, abdominal surgery is less painful and less costly. Patients have been known to spend only one day in the hospital after a laparoscopy; this means hospitals, insurers, employers and the patients save money.

Instead of having a large six- or 10-inch scar which would have been evident with the traditional method, all patients now have to show are four ballpoint-sized marks on the abdomen.

Dr. Michael O. Akpata, of Canada, who has successfully performed over 240 laparoscopic procedures, conducted the physician training at the seminar.

CIRCON-ACMI of California, provided the high-tech instrumentation to be used for procedures. It is the largest USA producer of medical endoscope and video systems. The company is a world leader in endoscopic innovation and design.

Endoscopic sales manager for AN-MED International conducted product briefings and served as coordinator of the event.

AN-MED International is a Florida-based medical export company that serves as the distributor for CIRCON-ACMI products in the Caribbean region.

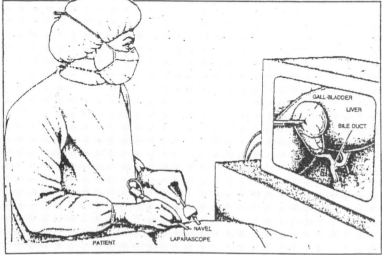

THE LAPAROSCOPE makes it possible for surgeons to remove diseased gall-bladders without having to open up patients' abdomens.

An article from *The Nation Sunday Sun* describing the new laparoscopic procedure, allowing gall bladder removal with a quicker recovery time.

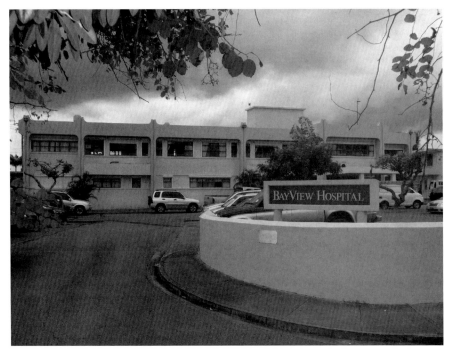

Bayview Hospital, Barbados.

which is another aspect of care available to the local population. Many minor issues can be dealt with in these clinics which usually include a pharmacy. It also helps the locals who depend on buses for transportation to be serviced in their own neighborhood.

During another one of my visits to the island, I was requested to teach some of the surgeons laparoscopic hernia repair. However, over time the surgeons who participated in this program found the procedure very tedious and time-consuming and therefore decided to stick with the old method of open hernia repair.

On one of our holidays to Barbados, I received a call from one of the general surgeons who had previously attended my laparoscopic teaching courses. Somehow he found out that I was on the island.

"Mike, glad to have you back on the island. Hope you are enjoying yourself. How would you like to come down to Bayview for a couple of hours and help me with a case?"

Prior to leaving for vacation I was exhausted from my workload in Windsor and was looking forward to swimming, reading and just generally relaxing.

One of the crew members on a Caribbean cruise ship had developed an incarcerated inguinal hernia which means that the hernia contents were bulging out and could not be pushed back into the groin. If left untreated this could cause strangulation of the hernial structures due to lack of blood supply.

He informed me that the patient required urgent surgery. He did not want the open method which would require too much time off work and the ship was scheduled to leave the following day.

The surgeon had suggested laparoscopy as another option and was happy to hear that I was in town. His experience was limited in this area and he was hoping that I would be able to guide him through the case. I hesitated for a moment as I was anxious to go to the beach but finally realized that it would not take too much away from my vacation.

When I arrived at the hospital, I examined the patient who appeared to be in a lot of pain. I discussed the pros and cons of laparoscopic inguinal hernia repair with him and had him sign the hospital consent. I also explained that if any complications arose, I might have no choice but to resort to an open method of treatment. I was able to perform his left inguinal hernia repair laparoscopically without any complications. My assistant and camera man during the surgery was the general surgeon who had requested my help.

Once the patient was transferred to the recovery room, I went into the doctor's lounge to change into my street clothes and leave the hospital. As I came out, I was met by the surgeon who thanked me and then handed me an envelope. I really did not mind helping out and was not expecting payment. I was later told that the patient did well and had sent a letter of gratitude to the hospital.

Whenever we go to Barbados on holidays, we always stop at Bayview Hospital to have a chat with the operating room staff as we have made many friends down there.

CHAPTER TWENTY SEVEN
OTHER PIONEERING INNOVATORS

Although I feel that I have contributed to the innovation of general surgery and gastrointestinal endoscopy during my years in Windsor, some of my colleagues, both surgeons and medical specialists, also promoted new procedures in their respective fields.

I will mention a few who I have been in contact with over the years most of them at Windsor Western. This is by no means a complete list of contributors to surgical innovations in this city but does show the talent and expertise that the citizens in Windsor have been blessed to have available to them.

I have approached all of the following who have given me permission to include their names and have provided an outline of their work for me.

DR. ISMAIL PEER

Dr. Peer first arrived in Canada in 1967 and started his practice in Windsor in 1972. He is a trained medical internist with a sub-specialty in gastroenterology and endoscopy and had privileges in all four hospitals in the city. He also was one of the pioneers of endoscopy using a flexible scope.

He one of those who initiated the procedure called, ERCP, which is the examination of the common bile duct and pancreatic duct using a fiberoptic scope. The injection of dye rules out blockage of the ducts either by stones or cancer of the pancreas.

Dr. Peer and I were responsible for the care of patients admitted into the intensive care unit at Windsor Western because there were no trained intensivists in the city at that time. We both took courses and were able to supplement and complement each other in caring for these patients.

DR. FOUAD TAYFOUR

Dr. Tayfour, a well renowned ophthalmologist, established his practice in Windsor in 1988. He specialized in cataract and retinal surgery and was the first to bring retinal surgery to Windsor and Essex County. In 1988, he performed the first vitrectomy and retinal detachment at Windsor Western. In 1990, he performed cataract surgery using the phaco-emulsification procedure and in 1991, he became the first surgeon in Canada to perform cataract surgery under topical anesthesia.

Until that time, cataract surgery was quite tedious and involved a lengthy hospital stay. This new method allowed the patient to go home the same day. He also performed the first clear corneal incision for cataract surgery.

He established the Windsor Laser Eye Institute and has since been on the forefront of laser vision correction surgery.

Dr. Tayfour was the first surgeon in North America to perform Lasik in 1993. He continues to maintain a strong interest in advancing the development of new procedures and the application of new technologies to clinical ophthalmology practice. Windsor has become a destination for other surgeons to learn surgical techniques and hospital efficiency.

He has generously given back to the community over the years. Among other things, he has donated a million dollars to Windsor Regional Hospital to assist in renovating the Western campus into a user friendly rehabilitative facility and mental health wing. This was in gratitude for the support he received from this hospital when he first arrived in the city.

DR. GEORGE WONG

Dr. Wong received his fellowship in cardiology in Toronto in 1977 and located his practice in Windsor the same year. He introduced the use of the Swan-Ganz catheter for hemodynamic monitoring of the cardiovascular system in intensive care patients.

M-Mode echocardiogram was becoming the standard cardiology investigation in the mid 1970s. On one occasion, he had a 15 year-old girl referred to him who had had a stroke with suspicious cerebral embolism (blood clot in the brain).

This event made a great case to vie for equipment to help diagnose a patient.

Because Windsor Western was open to such a state of the art procedure, the hospital purchased a trans-thoracic echo machine. With this new technology, it was confirmed that the patient's embolism did indeed originate from the heart and was caused by an atrial-septal defect.

This phenomenon started the era of cardiac ultrasound in Windsor. About five to

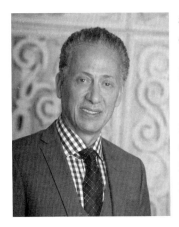

Dr. Fouad Tayfour.

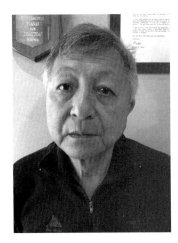

Dr. George Wong.

seven years later, trans-esophageal echocardiogram was introduced to Essex County.

In 1979, Dr. Wong accidentally discovered a coronary angiogram suite sitting idle in the x-ray department of Windsor Western which had previously been used by another invasive cardiologist who had practiced there before transferring to the United States.

With enormous support from the community, his peers and the hospital staff, Dr. Wong lobbied for the resurrection of the coronary angiogram program. The hospital had the foresight to recognize what a great service this would bring to the community.

Once a renowned cardiac surgeon in London had expressed satisfaction with the quality of the images and agreed to operate on those patients, the plan was put into motion.

Three to four years later, the community along with the Canadian Auto Workers (CAW) gave donations to Windsor Western helping to set up a new state of the art cardiac catheterization laboratory and the program was underway. The government formally recognized and funded the program.

In 1986, Dr. Wong started thrombolytic therapy using intravenous Streptokinase or TPA for patients experiencing acute myocardial infarction (heart attack). This treatment is critical in reducing heart muscle damage and increasing survival rates for people experiencing potential fatal events.

DR. RON SORENSEN

Dr. Sorensen is an urologist who has contributed extensively to the care of kidney patients in the Windsor area. While awaiting fellowship exams in 1982, he spent time with an astute specialist in interventional radiology in London and soon became adept with percutaneous renal access. By definition, this involves passing a tube through the skin (percutaneous) into the kidney for drainage or stone removal.

Normally urine from the kidney drains through a narrow muscular tube called the ureter into the bladder. Sometimes the tube is blocked by a stone or blood clot following trauma to the system. Other times, the obstruction may be due to cancer. The catheter which is inserted through the skin allows urine to drain from the kidney into a collecting bag outside the body.

The year after he began practice at Windsor Western, Dr. Sorensen attended a World Urology conference where Percutaneous Nephrolithotomy commonly known as 'Percs' was being discussed as the latest innovation. As there was no interventional radiologist at the hospital at that time, he was allowed to share the use of the Coronary Angiogram suite with Dr. Wong.

Dr. Sorensen became very adept at this procedure to the extent that during his first year in Windsor he successfully carried out 200 cases without the role of an interven-

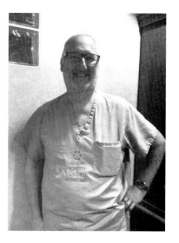

Dr. Ron Sorensen.

tional radiologist and had become known Canada wide for his expertise.

At the present time he has performed more than 3000 cases while teaching the procedure to some of the other urologists in the city.

Dr. Sorensen has been at the forefront of applying the latest innovations in the treatment of prostatic cancer either surgically or by the use of alternative procedures.

These have included the insertion of radiation seeds into the prostate called Brachytherapy done in conjunction with a radiation oncologist at Windsor Regional and cryotherapy (freezing of prostate tissue) which kills the cancer cells.

DR. BASSEL AL-FARRA

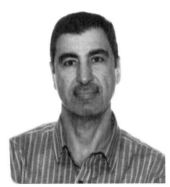

Dr. Bassel Al-Farra.

Dr. Al-Farra is another prominent urologist who has contributed to the advancement of urological surgery in Windsor. He attended the University of Toronto and moved to Windsor in 1990. In 1999, he instituted a new revolutionary technique which relieves urinary incontinence in women with the use of tension free vaginal tape surgery commonly called TVT.

A mesh tape is placed under the urethra like a sling or hammock to keep it in its normal position thereby providing support for the bladder so that any sudden cough or vigorous movement does not result in the accidental release of urine.

No large incision is involved as the tape is inserted through tiny incisions in the pelvic and vaginal wall. The operation takes about 30 minutes and is done under local anesthetic with sedation. At the end of the procedure, the patient is made to cough to make sure there is no leak.

There are several advantages to this procedure over the open method. They include quicker recovery time, no need for major surgery and minimal pain and discomfort post-operatively. There is usually no need to admit the patient into the hospital.

Dr. Al-Farra has done hundreds of these procedures with about a 98% success rate. Other urologists are now also using this method of TVT although not as frequently.

CHAPTER TWENTY EIGHT
HOSPITAL COMMITTEES

I was involved in several committees in the hospitals before they merged to two sites. Prior to amalgamation, my positions included the following:

GRACE HOSPITAL

• Pharmacy and Therapeutic Committee: We met once a month to discuss any matters pertaining to the introduction of new medications making sure that we were up to date in the treatment of patients. The financial aspect of the use of medications by physicians was also a common topic.

WINDSOR WESTERN HOSPITAL

• Intensive Care Committee: Dr. I. Peer and I were the primary physicians taking care of the patients in the intensive care unit. As mentioned before, there was no intensivist at the hospital. Dr. Peer was an internist with gastroenterology training and I was a general surgeon with endoscopic training. The work load allowed us to supplement and complement each other while caring for the patients in the unit.

• Tissue and Audit Committee: Usually there were six members on this committee including two general surgeons, one pathologist, one gynecologist, a general practitioner and an endocrinologist. The chairman of the committee when I first joined was Dr. Raphael Cheung.

Our mandate was to review all the surgical deaths and any unusual surgical and medical cases that had occurred in the hospital. If the members of the committee were satisfied that appropriate care had been rendered to the patients, no action was taken. However, if there was any concern by members of the committee, that particular chart was sent to the appropriate department of the primary care physician to be discussed. It was a useful committee for the hospital and ensured good patient care.

In 1991, I was elected as the head of the committee until amalgamation with Metropolitan Hospital.

HÔTEL DIEU HOSPITAL

• Medical Records Committee: This committee looked into the Admission and Discharge procedures of patients. This also included the review of the admission history and discharge summary to ensure that it was appropriate.

• Library Committee: Our job was to review the latest literature and decide which new text books would be appropriate to add to the library collection.

CHAPTER TWENTY NINE
SECRETARY TO THE DEPARTMENT OF SURGERY

In 1988, Dr. Charles Pearce, an urologist, was elected to the position of Chief of Surgery at Hôtel Dieu. Dr. Richard Anderson was elected as Deputy Chief and I was appointed to the position of Secretary. There was a lot of co-operation between us and we worked very well together as a team sharing the duties and responsibilities.

My role as secretary was to record the minutes of the meetings of the department of surgery and then send copies to each subsection of surgery. The department functioned in an exemplary manner. During my tenure, I initiated some new committees and resurrected some old ones.

• Death review committee: We had a monthly review of all surgical deaths occurring in the hospital. The meeting was usual-

Dr. Charles Pearce, past Chief of Surgery at Hôtel-Dieu Hospital.

ly held at 7 am with myself, Dr. Anderson, a third surgeon who has since left the city and Dr. Pearce as the chairman. The aim of this committee was to make sure that all surgical death reviews were transmitted to the individual sub-sectional chiefs for discussion within their department.

The purpose was not to cast aspersions on the integrity of the surgeon involved but rather to ensure that the care being provided to patients in the hospital was acceptable. In this regard, we also reviewed any unusual surgical misadventures in the operating room during surgery.

- Annual Surgical Dinner: This was a new program which I initiated. The idea first came to my attention during one of my surgical conferences in Spain and I thought this would be a good idea for our hospital in Windsor.

I approached Frank Bagatto, CEO of Hôtel Dieu, about the idea of sponsoring an annual surgical dinner during which time I would invite a specialist to discuss an important current topic with the entire department of surgery.

To my surprise we reached an agreement, the hospital would pay the guest speaker and also provide the food and drinks which would be served by the hospital staff. This dinner was to be held once a year at the end of June.

On this basis, we prepared for our first annual surgical dinner. I was responsible for choosing the topic and the speaker who I contacted personally. It was also my role to arrange for the transportation and accommodations and to introduce the speaker at the dinner meeting. In these events, I had the full cooperation of the CEO and his assistants.

The topic for the first annual surgical dinner was "Trauma and Critical Care Management" given by Dr. Girotti.

The next year, the topic of discussion was the introduction of laparoscopic cholecystectomy. At that time, I had taken this course and had already started courses in advanced laparoscopic procedures.

Again, I invited Dr. Girotti to be the guest speaker because by then he was the director of the laparoscopic teaching program for the University of London. He discussed this new surgical innovation using video presentation to emphasize his points. Many general surgical colleagues were so impressed with his talk that they applied for training in laparoscopic cholecystectomy.

The third topic for our annual meeting was the role of gastroenterology in G.I. surgery. Dr. Norman Marcon, Chief of Gastroenterology, Wellesley Hospital, Toronto and Associate Professor, University of Toronto, was our guest speaker. Dr. Marcon is renowned as a gastroenterologist and teacher in this field. This time, the gastroenterologists were also invited to the dinner as I knew they would benefit from the information provided as this was their field. Dr. Marcon discussed not only the features

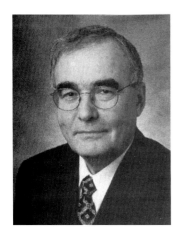

Frank Bagatto, former President and CEO of Hôtel-Dieu Hospital.

of gastroenterology but also the new innovations of therapeutic endoscopy. The talk was well received by all members present.

Our fourth meeting was on urological procedures. The speaker was Dr. Ray H. Littleton, head of Endo-Urology at Henry Ford Hospital in Detroit, Michigan. He was invited by our Chief of Surgery, Dr. Pearce. Among Dr. Littleton's topics was the use of flexible fiber optic scopes for cystoscopy and many other urological procedures rather than using the former rigid scope.

The fifth meeting topic was Laparoscopy in Trauma with Dr. Demetrius Litwin who was my mentor in Saskatoon for laparoscopic cholecystectomy and several other advanced laparoscopic procedures. Prior to moving to Toronto, he was the chief of laparoscopic surgery at Saskatoon City hospital. He later became professor of minimal invasive surgery, University of Toronto, Mount Sinai Hospital, for two years. Following this, he was appointed to the same position at the Massachusetts General Hospital, Cambridge, Massachusetts, which is part of the Harvard Medical School.

His speech was impressive and well received indeed, bearing in mind that laparoscopic surgery was only a few years into its development. Shortly after his visit, I had the opportunity to use this procedure on a motor vehicle accident victim with blunt intra-abdominal trauma at Windsor Western.

In 1995, we had our last surgical dinner meeting. The topic was Laparoscopic Spinal Surgery given by Dr. Isador Lieberman, an orthopedic surgeon at Toronto Western Hospital.

Present at the meeting were many surgeons, especially orthopedic surgeons and neuro surgeons who were based at Hôtel Dieu. In addition, we also invited the operating room nurses from both Hôtel Dieu and Windsor Western since the surgery was being performed at both sites.

Dr. Stephen Bartol and I had previously attended a hands-on course at Toronto Western Hospital under the directorship of Dr Lieberman. We were accompanied by two operating room nurses from Windsor Western who were taught the instrumentation and set-up from a nursing point of view. The neuro surgeons at Hôtel Dieu had just started this procedure but needed experienced laparoscopic general surgeons to complement them in the performance of anterior spinal surgery. Only those with advanced laparoscopic experience could pursue this course and for the most part included myself and Dr. Richard Anderson.

In the end, I felt a lot had been accomplished for the benefit of our patients in Windsor. It had been a very successful endeavor which would not have been possible without the effort, support and generosity of the CEO of Hôtel Dieu, who had agreed to support this new venture.

CHAPTER THIRTY
CHANGES IN DEPARTMENT OF SURGERY - HÔTEL DIEU

In 1993, Dr. Richard Anderson was appointed to the position of Chief of Surgery and I was both the Deputy Chief of Surgery and Secretary for the department. In this new position, I carried on with my previous duties. In addition, there were times that I acted as Chief of Surgery when Dr. Anderson was occasionally not available.

By this time, the amalgamation between Salvation Army Grace Hospital and Hôtel Dieu was taking place. This eventually led to the demise of the Annual Surgical Dinner meetings and the Death Review committee.

Once Dr. Anderson resigned as the Chief of Surgery, the new Chief of Staff appointed another surgeon as interim Chief of Surgery until elections could take place. In December of 1997, Dr. Robert Yovanovich, a senior orthopedic surgeon, was elected as the new Chief of Surgery.

I was elected to the position of head of the section of General Surgery and was asked to continue as Secretary to the Department of Surgery. In this capacity, I participated in the following committees:

• Tissue and Audit Committee: Now I was able to reintroduce the Tissue and Audit Committee to the hospital. It incorporated all sections of the department including general surgery, orthopedics, urology, and cardiovascular surgery.

I was the chairman of the committee and we met at 7 am on the first Friday of each month. I requested that the Medical Records Department provide me with the charts of surgical patients with unusual occurrences and the deaths from the various departments to be discussed at the meeting.

I would then hand out these charts to members of the committee to review individually before the monthly meeting. Any charts that the committee felt to be of concern would be passed on to the head of the department involved to be further discussed at their monthly meetings.

"This time I was able to convince the Chief of Neurosurgical Sciences to join the group for the first time."

• Clinical Pathology Conference: The role of the conference was to discuss any particular chart which the Tissue and Audit Committee members felt was questionable. In each instance those present would usually include the surgeon in charge of the case, a subspecialty member involved in the case, the radiologist and the pathologist.

I was the chairman and introduced the case to be discussed. The surgeon would present the case from his point of view and then the rest of the panel would give their opinion followed by questions from the members of the audience. I came up with this idea from a conference which I had attended dealing with abnormal pathology in surgery and found it to be an extremely informative session from the educational standpoint.

Initially, the members were happy to have the opportunity to discuss these cases. Unfortunately, as time went on, there was a feeling among a few members that my aim was to single out a particular person whose case was to be discussed, even though this was not my intention at all.

My main aim was to allow all of us to discuss surgical problems with input from the various subspecialties including pathology and radiology. After a lot of thought, my decision was to discontinue this important program.

• Quality Assurance Committee: I was appointed to this committee by the former Chief of Staff following the amalgamation of the hospitals. The committee met at 12 noon on the first Tuesday of each month. Its mandate was to ensure that every section of the hospital had adequate funding for its equipment and supplies in order to carry out their responsibilities. This committee reported its findings to the Medical Advisory Committee of the hospital.

• Operating Room Committee: I had been a member of the committee since 1997, representing the interests of the Section of General Surgery. Our monthly meetings involved discussions including the allocation of operating times to each section within the Surgical Department, discussion of new equipment needed by each section and any other overall problems arising in the operating room.

As Head of the Department of General Surgery, it was my role to divide our allotted operating room time equitably among our members including the occasional extra time that became available at a moment's notice.

Secondly, the Emergency Room trauma call coverage was discussed by this committee and it was my responsibility to speak out on behalf of my department whenever there was a point of contention regarding this coverage.

In short, my responsibility was to represent the members of our group to ensure smooth running of the operating room. My mandate was for three years.

In January of 2000, I was re-elected unanimously for an additional three years. We functioned as a cohesive group.

CHAPTER THIRTY ONE
SENTINEL LYMPH NODE BIOPSY

In the late 1990's, I found there was a worldwide interest in the use of sentinel lymph node biopsy as part of the treatment for breast cancer. Up to this point a much more invasive procedure called radical axillary lymph node dissection was commonly used following the diagnosis of breast cancer. This involves removing most or all of the lymph nodes (glands) from the axilla of the affected side to determine if any nodes contain cancer cells thus increasing the risk of metastatic disease. The results of the pathology examination help determine the course of follow up treatment at the Cancer Clinic.

Axillary node dissection can have significant complications including pain, irritation, infection, limitation of shoulder movement and swelling of the arm from a collection of lymphatic fluid. This can occur in 6 to 30% of axillary node dissections. As a result, new and better methods were being discussed.

A sentinel lymph node biopsy or SLNB is a procedure in which this node is identified, removed and examined to determine whether breast cancer cells have spread to it already. The sentinel node is the first lymph node from which cancer cells are most likely to spread to other lymph nodes.

This has to be determined by the pathologist. Usually an injection of radioactive dye is used to locate the node before it can be removed.

In contrast to axillary lymph node dissection, sentinel lymph node biopsy is a minimally invasive procedure with minimal side effects. A positive sentinel lymph node indicates that the cancer has spread to this node and may also be present in other nearby nodes or regional lymph nodes as they are called. This would then require the removal of the entire system of lymph nodes in the armpit.

On the other hand, if the sentinel lymph node is negative, then no axillary lymph node dissection is required saving the patient from a more extensive surgery.

I attended several courses to learn this procedure at Hôtel Dieu Hospital in Québec City, then at Victoriaville Hospital also in Quebec in 1997.

I was intensely excited about this new innovation and brought it back to our general surgical group for discussion. There was a mixed reaction from our group as to the acceptance and feasibility of this procedure. This would involve a multidisciplinary approach including the surgeon, the pathologist and the nuclear radiologist who would help determine the site of the sentinel lymph node.

This procedure was also one of the main topics of discussion at the Postgraduate Course, Toronto General Hospital, held on June 15-16, 2006 and June 12-13, 2008. I attended both.

CHAPTER THIRTY TWO
AMALGAMATION OF THE WINDSOR HOSPITALS

The original four hospitals were; Hôtel Dieu run by the Sisters of St. Joseph, Grace run by the Salvation Army, Metropolitan and finally Windsor Western commonly called IODE (Independent Order of the Daughters of the Empire) both city hospitals.

There was a lot of discussion about the union of these four hospitals some of which was very heated. Originally my main interest was at Windsor Western as I had the most available operating time there and to some extent Hôtel Dieu where I had more endoscopy time. The government wanted to save some money by this merger. I was not sure this was a good idea in the long run.

I was one of the few people who constantly opposed the idea of the merger on the following grounds:

• The city would be losing hospital beds, operating rooms and also emergency department facilities once the merger took place. In my opinion this would lead to a decrease in the provision of care to the patients.

• I was also concerned about the congestion that would take place in the two remaining hospitals and mounting delays in admitting patients.

• If the aim was for the provincial government to save money, it might have been more prudent to construct one large hospital in the city with all the adequate facilities under one roof. There was no guarantee that amalgamation would not cost more money because each of the two remaining hospitals required many more expensive renovations.

One of my suggestions was to keep the existing hospitals open with a division of services to each.

For example, Windsor Western could have been made into an ambulatory facility for same day surgeries such as cataracts, arthroscopy of joints and minor surgical procedures. There was plenty of space for parking and there would be no need for an emergency department.

Hôtel Dieu could have remained the main trauma center for the city. Metropolitan could have become a women and children's center as it is now and Grace could have been converted into long term care beds which are now desperately needed in the city.

In the end, the two religious hospitals were combined to form Hôtel Dieu-Grace Hospital, while the other two were combined to form Windsor Regional Hospital with two campus sites. Unfortunately, Grace Hospital was closed.

My feeling was that these final decisions had already been made long before any of the town hall meetings were arranged for input and discussion.

Another idea which I brought out was that the 'Walk-in Clinics' which were already opening around the city would be much more functional if they were strategically positioned and expanded to have several services under one roof. This would lessen the number of people required to attend the hospital emergency rooms and thus decrease waiting times for the critically ill. On top of that, hospitals would probably save money.

Many of the services were duplicated in all four hospitals and to some extent even when they were combined into two sites.

The cost of renovating these two older buildings has been quite high and we have lost many beds in the process.

CHAPTER THIRTY THREE
MCMASTER UNIVERSITY HEALTH SCIENCES

McMaster University Health Sciences under the directorship of Dr. Mehran Anvari set up a Center for Minimal Access Surgery (CMAS) as part of its continuing Medical Education program.

Advanced laparoscopic surgery took a great leap forward with the opening of this new center. It became the lightning rod that propelled both the recently taught surgeons and those like myself who had participated in numerous courses and had some experience in laparoscopic surgery.

Dr. Anvari is quite an aggressive and efficient surgeon and as an instructor made these difficult surgical advances available to all surgeons across Canada. I attended many of the courses under his supervision and each time I learned a new technique to assist me in my quest to achieve excellence in laparoscopic surgery.

My first course at the CMAS was on March 24-25, 2000. It involved anti-reflux surgery which is called laparoscopic Nissen fundoplication to prevent the reflux of food, acid and bile in the stomach from backing up into the esophagus or lungs. We also learned how to become more proficient at suturing and tying knots laparoscopically.

During the summer of 2000, I was made aware that Dr. Anvari had eight cases of Nissen fundoplication booked in the operating room for the same day. I thought this would be a perfect opportunity for me to stay with him for the entire day watching the same procedure over and over learning by repetition and being able to ask any questions that might arise. At the end of these procedures, I was exhausted.

I knew that I had a long drive back to Windsor and that I was booked for surgery the following morning at Windsor Western. Staying overnight in Hamilton was not an option.

I decided that I would try to drive home that same evening taking several breaks along the way.

When I got out onto Highway 401, there were a lot of transport trucks on the road. I had classical music on the radio and my travel was progressing well. I followed behind one of the trucks for quite a distance until I was back in Essex County. That's when I started thinking about all the things I still had to do that evening when I got home.

I made the horrible mistake of deciding to pass him and several other trucks that were lined up in front of him. I was trying to keep my distance from the truck and must have pulled too far to the left as I was passing him, hitting the gravel edge near the median.

Suddenly, I felt my car curve to the edge of the road on the right and I was thrown into the air. I could feel my car spinning. Then I felt the car somersaulting and thought my life was over.

I did not panic. I actually felt at peace.

My car landed on the opposite side of the road on the trunk and gradually dropped forwards onto all four wheels. The car was a total wreck and I was stunned and trapped inside.

From the ditch I saw a FedEx van speeding towards me. The driver and three other men suddenly appeared. I tried to climb out of my car but I could not.

Then I heard one of them say, "Oh my God, it's Dr. Akpata. Quick, open the door."

With God on my side and the help of these compassionate men, I was able to get out of the car and roll onto the ground. I felt pain in both shoulders.

One of the men then called for an ambulance which arrived within minutes. I was rushed to the emergency department of Hôtel Dieu.

When I arrived, I noticed how quickly everyone was attending to me. The emergency doctor arranged to have x-rays done while some blood samples were being taken. I was given an intramuscular injection for pain. All in all, I was fairly stable.

At the end, there were no broken bones except that I had injured both of my shoulders and had a lot of generalized aches and pains. After all the tests were completed, I was admitted into the hospital for observation overnight and was fit to be released the following day.

I was able to walk out on my own and seeing how all of the important procedures were followed religiously, I thanked the entire staff for their life-saving efforts.

The four gentlemen, who were so kind to stop and help, were on their way to Toronto but stopped to phone the emergency department to find out how I was doing. I later learned, the one who recognized me at the scene of the accident was the son of a man whom I had previously operated on for cancer of the bowel.

I learned an important lesson from this experience. I would never again overextend myself for any training course and would always plan an extra day for travel.

The next course I attended at the CMAS involved advanced laparoscopic splenectomy (removal of spleen), bilateral adrenalectomy (removal of adrenal gland) and pancreatic surgery, on December 1-2, 2000. By this time, I had done almost every intra-abdominal surgical procedure laparoscopically with the exception of pancreatectomy for cancer of the pancreas.

Before, in 1993, I had removed an enlarged spleen (splenomegaly) in a young girl at Hôtel Dieu and published the results

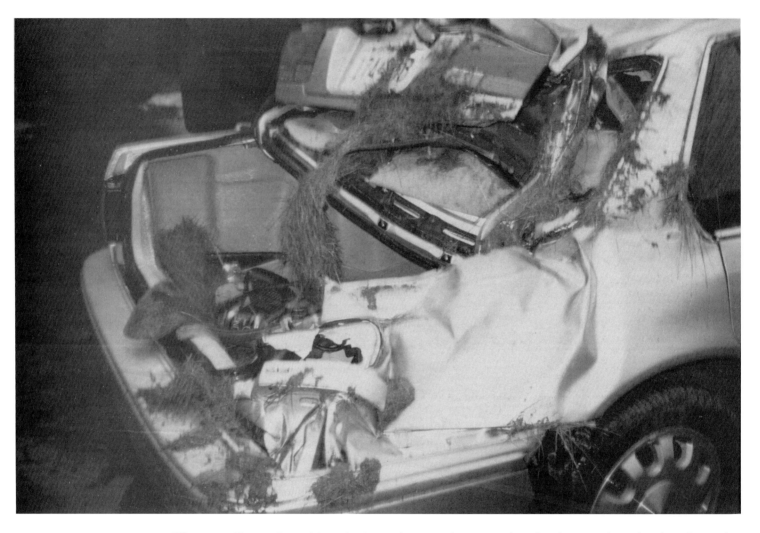
The car flipped and landed on the trunk, completely destroying the back end.

in the Canadian Journal of Surgery in February of 1995. The title of the publication was: 'Laparoscopic Splenectomy for Congenital Spherocytosis with Splenomegaly: a Case Report.' Reference CJS, Vol. 38, No.1, February 1995.

It was a unique case because the spleen was at least five times the normal size and it was extremely difficult to do it laparoscopically. With persistence and an excellent assistant I was able to complete the case and was quite pleased, hence the publication.

Adrenalectomy was another difficult case and I usually worked with one of the urologists. I did only a handful of them and did not publish any in the journals. The last procedure that I learned laparoscopically was the repair of an incisional ventral hernia and I must say that its outcome is far superior to the open method.

CHAPTER THIRTY FOUR
ENDOSCOPIC PRACTICE

As I am a general surgeon with extra training in endoscopy, a large part of my practice involved using a flexible scope to examine the gastrointestinal tract. Gastroscopy involves inserting a flexible tube into the mouth, through the esophagus, into the stomach and through the first part of the small bowel called the duodenum which is 10 to 12 inches long. Most often, biopsies are taken of any suspicious areas and also to check for the presence of the Helicobacter pylori organism which has been found in more recent years to be the cause of stomach ulcers.

Colonoscopy involves examination of the large bowel which is approximately 5 feet long, from the anus to the junction of the small bowel or terminal ileum. The small bowel in comparison is 20 to 23 feet long. Biopsies of any suspicious areas are taken and polyps are routinely removed and sent to pathology to rule out cancer.

Photographs of any unusual findings found in the entire gastrointestinal tract are taken in addition to the biopsies.

I had my first training in this procedure during my residency years at the University of Alberta and I was lucky enough to have private tutoring from a gastroenterologist at Mercy Hospital in Calgary, Alberta. When I arrived in Windsor, I applied for privileges in all four hospitals to perform both general surgery and G.I. Endoscopy.

Other than myself at that time, there was no other general surgeon in Windsor trained to use the new flexible endoscopes. Until that point all procedures were being done with a rigid metal scope. Dr. Peer was an internist performing these procedures using the flexible scope.

Although I was granted privileges in both specialties, I was requested to provide proof of proficiency in G.I. Endoscopy to maintain my privileges since it was an innovation in general surgery at the time. That's when I decided to undergo addition-

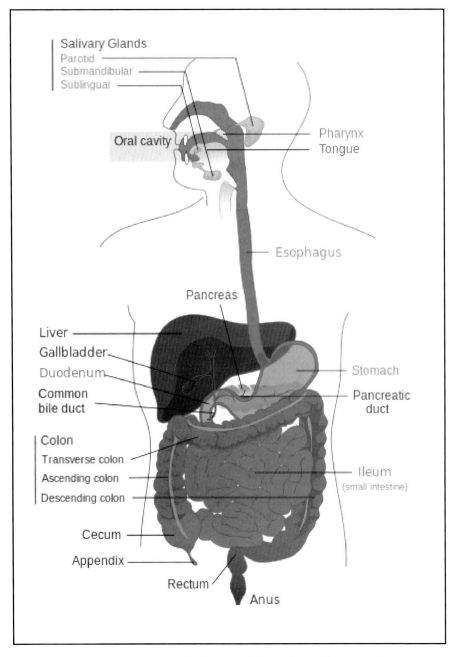

A chart of the digestive system.

al training in Toronto to satisfy the request of the Credentialing Committees.

I applied to Dr. Norman Marcon, Chief of the Division of Gastroenterology at Wellesley Hospital in Toronto, to undergo comprehensive endoscopy training under his directorship. This took place from December 3-6, 1979. In the meantime, I put my practice on hold in Windsor. Dr. Marcon would do his first procedure in the morning and then I would do the other cases under his supervision the rest of the day.

The cases included upper and lower gastrointestinal tract examination. The procedures involved biopsies of abnormal areas of the gut and polypectomy (removal of polyps) for examination. Among the diseases identified were diverticular disease (pockets formed from weakened areas in the bowel), ulcerative colitis (ulcerated areas in the large bowel) and Crohn's disease (a serious chronic inflammatory bowel disease with ulceration causing diarrhea containing blood, pus and mucous).

Dr. Marcon found my hand-eye coordination to be excellent and the maneuvering of the scope to be satisfactory. Other gastroenterologists in Dr. Marcon's department participated in my supervision including Dr. Gregory Haber, Dr. Paul Kortan and Dr. M. S. Thirumurthi of Women's College Hospital. Dr. Haber and I did numerous cases together starting early in the morning and sometimes working until 8 pm.

Following the course, each of them agreed that I was well qualified to carry out endoscopic procedures in conjunction with my general surgery. Dr. Marcon sent a letter of recommendation on my behalf to the Credentials Committee of Hôtel Dieu dated December 6, 1979 with copies to the other hospitals.

During this session in Toronto, I also spent some time at Rudd Clinic, where I carried out colonoscopies with Dr. Rudd as the preceptor. In his letter to the Credentials Committees of all four hospitals, he indicated that I had demonstrated considerable skill in the technique of colonoscopy.

With the roadblocks cleared, I was able to start my surgical practice in January of 1980 to include endoscopy at all four Windsor hospitals. The advantage of a surgeon performing the endoscopic procedure is that he has visually seen the exact position of the tumor, making it easier to locate the site at the time of surgery.

I decided to attend additional gastrointestinal endoscopic clinics whenever I could. On March 14-15, 1980, I attended the Continuing Medical Education Seminar studying colonoscopy at the Cleveland Clinic, Ohio. Emphasis was placed on the need for slow withdrawal of the scope in order not to miss any polyps which can hide in the folds of the bowel.

Eventually, several other gastroenterologists came to the city and as a group we set up endoscopic seminars on a monthly basis where we had the opportunity to discuss new techniques and treatment of diseases of the gastrointestinal tract. These seminars qualified for credits at the Royal College of Physicians and Surgeons of Canada.

After five years of practice, I decided that it would be a good idea to undergo a refresher course in G.I. Endoscopy as the volume of my work in that area was increasing exponentially. I approached Dr. Norman Marcon again to accept me for another period of preceptorship.

This took place from January 8-18, 1985 inclusive. We went through some of the more difficult cases that he had. He emphasized repeatedly that the withdrawal time of the colonoscope should not be less than 6 minutes ensuring not to miss small polyps on the way out. This was the same recommendation that had been made at my previous course in Cleveland.

It is interesting to note that 10 years later, this aspect of withdrawing the colonoscope was emphasized by the Canadian Association of General Surgeons and the Journal of Gastroenterology. Those two weeks of training provided me with a wealth of information and experience.

Eventually, there was an influx of gastroenterologists and a larger number of general surgeons with privileges in endoscopy, which began to limit the allotted time available for each of us to carry out these procedures. This situation was made even worse by the amalgamation of the four hospitals into two resulting in my loss of endoscopic time at Grace and Windsor Western hospitals. A program was later set up at Hôtel Dieu–Grace Hospital whereby Friday afternoon was set aside strictly for screening colonoscopies on a rotational basis among the group.

In spite of the additional half day every two months for screening colonoscopy, my own personal waiting list was still very high. I approached Rosemary Lemmon, Director of the Operating Room at Leamington District Memorial Hospital, to see if there was any additional time available for endoscopy procedures. I learned there were some random days available which were then offered to me.

Eventually a system was worked out by Dr. Ejaz Ghumman, Chief of Surgery, who gave me every Monday for endoscopy in return for emergency surgical coverage one weekend per month. Also, one of the surgeons was moving to the Caribbean which made more operating time available.

Fortunately, most of my Windsor patients did not mind the trip to Leamington as it meant they would be able to get their procedure done more quickly. Needless to say, I utilized this extra time to the fullest by doing anywhere from 16 to 20 procedures per day. This helped me tremendously to clear my backlog of endoscopy patients.

The operating room staff at this hospital was very supportive and appreciative of my work. I continued to work there for three years from 2006 to 2009.

Although the extra work at Leamington Hospital increased my stress load, I felt I had done what was necessary for my patients.

CHAPTER THIRTY FIVE
PLANS FOR PRIVATE ENDOSCOPY CLINIC

In 2004, I attempted to set up a private endoscopic clinic in Windsor for myself and my associates. I always felt that this was the way of the future.

I met with a retired general surgeon who was one of the owners of such a clinic during a clinical symposium in Toronto. His clinic was doing well in spite of the fact that he was charging his patients a professional fee in addition to the amount paid by the Ontario Health Insurance Plan. This did not dissuade people as they could get the test done much sooner than in the hospitals and in a private setting.

I gave this new incentive a lot of thought and then decided to approach professionals in the field to help me with the logistics of setting up an endoscopy clinic here in Windsor. I was put in contact with his clinic administrator and accountant who explained in great detail the process involved.

A second meeting was arranged with several of my colleagues, both surgeons and gastroenterologists, to discuss these details with the administrative staff. At the time there was space available in my office complex which could have been developed into a clinic setting. The plan was generally thought to be a good idea until it came time to discuss the overall cost factor of setting up and furnishing this clinic and what each person would be responsible for contributing.

It was suggested that each patient would have to pay a fee of approximately $150 over and above what OHIP would pay to make it a viable plan. The general consensus was that it would be hard to find enough people willing to pay the extra fee in Windsor and that most of us were not business minded. Everyone had hospital privileges and could get full payment for procedures and not have to worry about overhead costs.

I was disappointed that the plan fell through because this was a new concept in Windsor and not without drawbacks.

The idea of an endoscopy unit outside of the hospital setting was still in my mind as a viable option. I even investigated the small operating theater that Dr. Tayfour had set up in his building for private patients. After lengthy discussions, it was again decided that this would not be a feasible option for our purposes.

Towards the end of 2009, having worked for over 30 years in a state of constant pressure from the commitment to my job, I was beginning to feel that the time had come to slow down and change my lifestyle. It was as if I was burning the candle at both ends and I was concerned that additional stress might lead to a physical ailment.

I requested from our group to take half of the emergency calls in return for giving up half of my operating and endoscopy time. Meanwhile, my practice was still increasing especially for endoscopy and there was inadequate time allotment at Hôtel Dieu-Grace for the number of patients that I had waiting. This was partially due to the fact that screening colonoscopy was now recommended by the government for early detection of colon cancer.

I decided that the time had come to gradually slow down in my overall practice of general surgery and endoscopy.

In September of 2009, I was approached by the business manager of a proposed endoscopic clinic in Windsor to consider joining their team. The owner of this new clinic also had a plastic surgery clinic and an endoscopy suite in Sarnia, Ontario.

I told him that I would think about it as I was in the process of slowing down my surgical practice but still had a backlog of endoscopy patients waiting.

By December 2009, I had made up my mind to retire from Hôtel Dieu-Grace, close my surgical practice but continue with my endoscopic practice at Leamington Hospital. I met several times with both the owner of the clinic and his business administrator to discuss the progress of the building site and the proposed working agreement.

After considering all the possibilities, I decided that working here on a part-time basis would be the best way to gradually retire. He was happy to accept me as part of his staff. The clinic was scheduled to be completed by January of 2010, however, as expected with any construction project, there were many delays resulting in the clinic opening in mid April. Just as in the hospital, the Ontario Health Insurance Plan (OHIP) covered all costs to the patient. My income was an agreed upon percentage of the daily procedures which I performed.

This was considerably less than the income from my endoscopic practice at the hospital but was also a way to gradually slow down and stop practice altogether. I was asked to start on a more full-time basis, that is, four days a week beginning at 8 am and ending at 5 pm on a temporary basis until another endoscopist was found to share the work load. I decided to give this plan a try.

Meanwhile, staff was being recruited including a Registered Nurse and many RNAs trained in endoscopic services. I recommended my office secretary, Carol, to the owner of the clinic as being highly efficient, dedicated to her work and able to deal well with the public. She was hired to help set up the office, handle bookings and prepare for patients.

CHAPTER THIRTY SIX
AN UNEXPECTED EVENT

I had booked a vacation to Barbados that same year to return April 17 as the clinic was scheduled to open on the 19. While in the departure lounge of the Barbados airport, I went to the washroom just before boarding the plane. To my surprise, I noticed blood in the toilet bowl after passing my urine. Prior to this experience, I had never had this problem in my life.

I was flabbergasted and scared.

As you can imagine, it was one of the longest rides home as my mind was racing from one diagnosis to the other. I had no pain which pretty much discounted a kidney stone. I became quite concerned also as the clinic was scheduled to open Monday morning and all the staff were in place. But then, after the first episode of bleeding, it disappeared for about a week.

On April 19, 2010 as planned, I attended my first day at the clinic and I was feeling physically fit but still concerned about the incident which had just occurred at the airport. The facilities in the clinic were satisfactory and every member of staff was happy to be there. At this point I was working every day but Wednesdays when I had my own office hours.

Initially, I started doing 13 procedures a day including both upper and lower gastrointestinal endoscopy, but gradually the number rose to about 17 and sometimes more.

At the end of the day, arrangements were made for me to do follow-up on any patients who had biopsies taken or polyps removed. I would discuss my findings with them and suggest any appropriate medication or life style changes to improve their condition and send a follow-up note to the family doctor.

Any biopsy or polyp removed which showed cancer was immediately referred to one of my colleagues in the hospital for further treatment.

My urologist friend, Dr. Bassel Al-Farra, continued investigations into the appearance of blood in the urine as it did recur from time to time. On one occasion during a weekend, he performed a cystoscopy with injection of dye into the kidneys. The radiologist felt that there was something suspicious in the left kidney which should be further investigated.

I then decided that for privacy reasons, I would feel more comfortable if I was transferred to the urological group in London. Dr. Al-Farra was willing to refer me to a specialist there.

A biopsy of the area in question was done and it showed that cancer was in its early stages in the kidney.

An operation to remove the left kidney was carried out on September 24, 2010 by Dr. Joseph Chin, who is well known and respected across Canada. My post operative care was excellent and I was discharged home within a week.

It is now over three years since my surgery and I have had no problems whatsoever.

I am sincerely grateful to all the specialists involved, including the radiologists at Windsor Regional and Hôtel Dieu-Grace for their commitment to my medical problem. Finally, I thank God for being so kind to me and guiding the hands of those involved in my care.

As part of the recovery from my surgery, I decided to spend some time in Barbados. This holiday gave me the opportunity to critically assess my future plan for my professional life as a whole and especially my commitment to the Windsor endoscopy clinic. So I could make an accurate decision, I wrote down the pros and cons of continuing with the clinic even at a slower pace, reviewed my health situation and took into account my personal experiences professionally and finally my family's concerns about me.

When I discussed the situation with my family both here and abroad, the answer was the same everywhere. All were concerned about my health and welfare and felt it was time for me to take care of myself and learn to enjoy the beauty around me.

Now was the time to take my request to God and ask for His direction.

The message was loud and clear that I should listen to all concerned with my welfare and retire from medicine. There is no doubt that anxiety and worry contributed to my ill health. On my return from holidays, I told the clinic director that I was no longer going to continue working there, ending my career in medicine.

I knew that I would miss it tremendously.

CHAPTER THIRTY SEVEN
GOOD SAMARITANS IN MY LIFE

One of my favorite sports since I was a student at King's College, was the game of squash which I played practically every day. It is such a good sport that a player needs only about 45 minutes of play time to have a good work-out.

When I arrived in Canada in 1960, I continued playing throughout my university years and eventually when I moved to Windsor I joined the Windsor Indoor Club where I played regularly. In addition to the physical aspect, I have met some trusted friends through this sport over the years.

During one of these squash tournaments, I was hit in my right eye by a fast returning ball. I fell down and for a brief second everything went dark. I had lost my vision. My sight returned within 15 to 30 seconds but I knew that I had to go the emergency department for examination and treatment.

The physician on call felt there was no serious injury to my eye so I put on my pair of dark glasses and went home. The following day, I was quite concerned when my right eye became more painful and I could see shadows crossing my vision on that side.

I contacted Dr. Tayfour and told him what had happened. After examining my eyes, he informed me that I had a small retinal tear in my right eye.

Without hesitation, he booked me for a special procedure called cryotherapy to be done the next day in his office. After the procedure, he told me to wear dark glasses on the way home because my eye had been dilated and would be affected by the sunlight.

Within a few days, the sight in my right eye had returned to normal. I was very grateful to him for his care for without good vision I could not continue in my capacity as a surgeon.

In April of 2003, I booked off two weeks to relax and recuperate in Barbados from my busy schedule. The sun and beaches were calling me but a couple of days before we left the city, I noticed a nagging pain in my right thigh. When it was time to fly from Toronto to Barbados, I was so incapacitated with pain that I had to be taken on board the plane in a wheelchair. I did not think much of this being a serious problem as I knew that I would be getting plenty of rest once we were settled at our destination.

I attributed the pain to my job which involved prolonged periods of standing and bending forward during laparoscopy and endoscopy and I thought that with rest from my work the pain would dissipate.

Over the next few days, however, the pain continued unabated. I decided to see, Dr. Jerry Thorne, a friend of mine who was an orthopedic surgeon at Bayview Hospital. After examination, he informed me that I should have an MRI done.

This was to ensure that there was no serious problem involving my back as disc disease sometimes radiates pain to the leg. He informed me that this would cost between $2500 to $3000 Barbados which is equivalent to about $1500 US.

I decided the best course of action was to return home earlier than planned and have any x-rays and treatment in Windsor. He prescribed some pain medication for me and I made arrangements with Air Canada to change my flight plans.

I left Barbados on April 26, 2003. The following morning, I called my family doctor who suggested that I go to the emergency department for examination. I was driven there by a friend and examined by an internist who requested x-rays of my spine and pelvis and felt that a CT scan of the spine would also be helpful.

Once the procedures were carried out, I came home and contacted my good friend, Dr. Chakravarthi, a well known neurosurgeon at Hôtel Dieu–Grace. I related my problems to him and that is when he took over the role of what I call a 'Good Samaritan'.

The following day he came to my house to examine me. I was alone and struggling to get out of bed when I realized that I was unable to walk. I was forced to crawl.

He insisted on making us both a cup of tea while I described my ordeal. When the tea was finished, he left the house and said, "I will be right back."

Within a few minutes, he came back and said, "I am taking you to the hospital and it looks like you will require surgery tonight. You probably have a prolapsed disc and the sooner we remove it the less chance you have of developing paralysis of the right leg."

Meanwhile, he had flattened out one of the seats in his van for me to lie on for the trip to the hospital. I was mesmerized that he was willing to do this for me.

First he made me a cup of tea, secondly, he offered to drive me to the hospital and thirdly, he was willing to carry out spinal surgery on me the same day. I was impressed by his friendship and kindness.

Dr. Chakravarthi took me straight to the emergency department and booked me for an MRI which confirmed the diagnosis of a prolapsed disc in my lower back at the L4-L5 position. From there he went to the Admitting Department to take care of all the paperwork and since I was a member of staff, he requested a private room.

None were available at that time but the admitting secretary suggested a palliative care room which was presently unoccupied.

While all these arrangements were being made, Dr. Chakravarthi went to the operating room to book me for my surgery. Unfortunately, the operating room was quite busy that evening and rather than starting my case in the later hours, I was booked for first thing the next morning. This whole affair was beyond my comprehension.

The following morning I was taken to the operating room. A lot of the nurses and other staff members were surprised to see me and came over to wish me well. As I was being wheeled into the theater, I said a silent prayer for God to guide my surgeon's hands. When I woke up after the surgery, I was relaxed and peaceful.

My post operative management and care was exemplary. During the recuperative phase I was dedicated to the instructions and exercises provided to me and was able to gradually return to work. Several nurses from the operating and recovery room welcomed me back with group photos.

I have never had a problem with my back since that time unlike many others who continue to suffer pain and debilitation after surgery.

I shall always be grateful to 'Chak' for his special care and surgical expertise.

I will never forget these two men who played a very important role in my health care. Each of these incidents could have resulted in the end of my surgical career if they had not been handled as quickly and efficiently as they were.

CHAPTER THIRTY EIGHT
HISTORY OF THE BENIN KINGDOM

I was born in Benin City, when Nigeria was still a British colony. The history of Benin City dates back to when it was the capital of a vast empire in West Africa covering about one fifth of present day Nigeria. It had great pre-eminence and recognition both in the whole of Africa and in Europe at that time. The Benin Kingdom should not be confused with the modern day country of Benin, formerly Dahomey, a previous French colony in West Africa.

The original founders of the Benin Empire, the Edo people, were ruled by Ogisos (Kings of the Sky) who eventually became known as Obas or kings. It is said to be one of the oldest sustained monarchies in the world. By tradition, the title of Oba or king goes to the eldest son.

By the 15th century, Edo or Benin, which originally was a group of protected settlements, was expanded into a thriving city-state. Under the 12th King called Ewuare the Great, the city-state was expanded into an empire. At that time, the city was actually called 'Ubinu or Bini' in the local mixed dialect. It was the Portuguese who first called it Benin City from this colloquial version which was later adopted by the locals.

The Oba or king had become the greatest power within the region. He was in command of a well organized, strong and disciplined army of men who were able to protect and expand the kingdom.

Beginning in about 800 A.D., the kings began to construct a series of walls around the city as a fortification against neighboring rivals. An inner earthen wall about 7 miles long was also built to enclose the palace grounds surrounded by a 50 foot deep moat.

According to the Guinness Book of World Records, the walls of Benin City were the second largest man-made structure after the Great Wall of China in terms of length. The series of earthen ramparts is the most extensive earthwork in the world.

Early Europeans were very impressed with the city's grandeur and level of organization comparing it to many other European cities of the time such as Lisbon, Antwerp, Madrid and Florence. The state had an advanced artistic culture and became famous for its artifacts in bronze, iron and ivory.

The first European travelers to reach Benin were the Portuguese explorers, in about 1485. A strong business relationship developed with tropical products such as ivory, pepper and palm oil being traded with the Portuguese for European goods such as manila and guns.

In the early 16th century, the Oba sent an ambassador to Lisbon and the King of Portugal sent Christian missionaries to Benin City. Some residents of Benin City could still speak pigeon Portuguese in the late 19th century.

The first English expedition to the country was in 1553, and significant trading developed mainly based on the same exports of ivory, palm oil and pepper. These traders in the 16th and 17th centuries brought back to Britain, tales of the 'Great Benin', a fabulous city of noble buildings ruled by a powerful king. However, the Oba began to suspect Britain of larger colonial designs and refused to sign their trade agreement.

This resulted in the British Expedition of 1896-97 when the British troops captured, burned, and looted the city of Benin. Many busts and portrait figures made of iron, carved ivory and particularly brass (known as the 'Benin Bronzes') were taken by the British and are now found in museums all over the world, especially in England.

This brought the Benin Empire to an end. Benin City is now as it was in the early years, the center of the rubber industry with cocoa plantations and also the centre for processing palm nuts into oil. As nature would have it, the first oil was found in Benin province many years later.

Over the years, millions of people have traveled to China to see the Great Wall as part of a world tour. A greater interest and more foresight in maintaining the original Benin City Walls could have resulted in a constant source of revenue both for Benin and Nigeria as a major tourist destination.

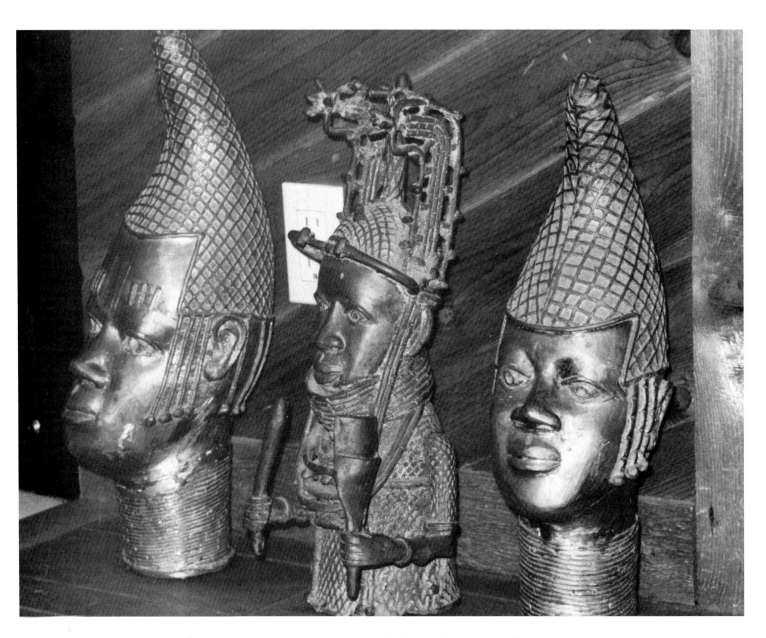

Benin bronzes belonging to Michael's cousin Sunny.

In my opinion, Nigeria has missed a great opportunity.

CHAPTER THIRTY NINE
FAMILY BACKGROUND

I was fortunate to have been born into the Akpata family in Benin City. The Akpata name is very well-known and respected in the area and has been influential over the years in the development of the city of Benin.

Many members of my extended family took part in the local administration of the city and province of Benin and also were involved in federal politics. Some were made local chiefs of the Benin Kingdom, including my father. It was in this environment in which I grew up prior to coming to Canada in 1960.

My grandfather was called Pa Okoro Akpata. He was a direct descendant of the ruling family of Usen which was one of the local government areas of the old Benin Kingdom. I did not have the opportunity to know him, but from the oral and written stories about him, he was a very successful man with high Christian values.

He and his brothers were hard working, well educated and attained a position of respect and leadership in the country. As I remember, he and his wife had six children, five sons including my father and one daughter.

My father was born on February 22, 1896 and became Chief Akitola Akpata before his death on June 28, 1980. He attended three elementary schools, Government School in Benin City, then two Christian boarding schools, St. David's School Akure and St. Savior's School in a town called Ijebu-Ode. He was the first of many members of the Akpata family to attend the famous King's College in Lagos from 1915 to 1919.

My father worked at the Elder Dempster Shipping Agency in Lagos in 1920 - 1921 and was the principal agent for John Holt Limited, two very reputable British companies in Nigeria. He was highly regarded by both companies for the work he did. Following this, he started and ran the Akpata Transport Service which became the fore-runner of the Armels Transport Company, similar to the Greyhound bus service in Canada.

When my father was a second year student at King's College, the eldest son of the Oba of Benin was admitted into his first year. As in many educational institutions, a first year student is attached to a more senior student. In this case, my father was assigned to the Oba's son as his mentor.

He helped him in any way possible since both of them were from Benin. Following the death of his father, Oba Akenzua the First, this student became the next Oba of Benin, Oba Akenzua the Second. Due to his close relationship with my father, he subsequently made my father a prominent chief and confidant.

My father, one of the eight advisors surrounding the monarch, was later appointed to the position of Chief Tax Officer for the Benin Native Authority. With that, he also became a member of the town planning authority.

As part of his dedication to his Christian faith, he was a founding member of the U.N.A. (United Native African) Church Cathedral in Benin City. He was also the manager of the church's school from 1948 to 1951.

When we were young, we all attended St. Matthew's Anglican Church where my uncle was the organist.

Following in the steps of my grandfather, my father also developed his own business enterprises, including rubber, timber and cocoa plantations and exported to countries including Britain, Europe and Russia. This business was very successful.

Another aspect of his professional life involved his contribution to several major national newspapers on contemporary affairs and he was for some time the Chief Correspondent of the Daily Times newspaper in Benin City. The Daily Times was the main national newspaper with headquarters in the capital city of Lagos. It was always an experience every Friday to read his editorials on current political issues.

There is a special occasion in Benin City, called the Ugieoba Festival which lasts 7-10 days between December and January. It is a very spiritual time similar to Christmas and Hanukkah when prayers are offered for peace, love, joy, prosperity and harmony.

On a particular day, the citizens of the city would wake up early at about 5 am and run in groups past my father's house towards a demarcated forest enclave. Their aim was to harvest Ewere leaves from a special tree which supposedly carry a good omen. They sang and danced their way back to the city carrying these leaves past my father's house towards the Oba's palace, about four blocks away.

During that afternoon, it was my father's role as one of the chiefs to wear a special robe with extensive coral beads round his neck and waist, and a special hat also containing coral beads. This was in preparation for a regal dance from our house to the Oba's palace.

From my recollection, two special chiefs came early in the morning to assist him in getting dressed. Hundreds of followers then danced with my father along the street to traditional drum music. Because of the weight of the coral beads, he was always accompanied by two men who helped him walk.

At this point, the grounds of the King's palace would be crowded by celebrants, including the populace, other chiefs and of course the King, who would be seated on a throne outdoors in his ceremonial robes, surrounded by his numerous wives in regal clothing.

When it was my father's turn, he would dance around the square in front of the crowd and then approach the Oba with a specific tribal dance. This dance would include the tossing of a special tribal sword called 'Eben' catching it mid air several times.

This sword must never touch the ground or it was thought to bring bad luck.

The crowd would be ecstatic and clapping incessantly for both my father and the King. Following this, my father would dance close to the Oba and present the Ewere leaves to be distributed among the dignitaries present.

At the end of the dance, my father would raise his right hand in a fist and touch his outstretched left hand, raising it towards the Oba in a traditional way of paying respect. This would be the end of my father's role in performing the Ugie dance.

He was the only chief assigned to perform this part of the festival since his title was the Ayobahan of Benin.

The King would climax the ongoing festival by blessing his people and his land before attending a Thanksgiving service at his regular church the following day. This ceremony still goes on today.

CHAPTER FORTY
FAMILY UPBRINGING

As well as being very religious, my father followed the traditional native law and customs allowing him to have more than one wife. My mother was the youngest of the three in the household at that time. Due to circumstances of which I am unaware, she left our home after having three children. I was the eldest.

I was about five years old when she left and we remained in the care of our father and two step-mothers. We also had a cook to help prepare the meals for our family. I spent most of my younger years in boarding schools and did not have much contact with my mother until shortly before she died at the age of forty-three from a stomach illness.

I had just completed my medical training at the University of Alberta in June 1966 when I decided to take my wife home to introduce her to my family. It was also an opportunity for me to visit my mother in the hospital. I was notified of her death by telegram December 29, 1966.

Altogether my father had twelve children, seven boys and five girls. He insisted that we take our education seriously and so he made it his priority to send most of us to a boarding school. He was pleased when several of us ultimately became profession-

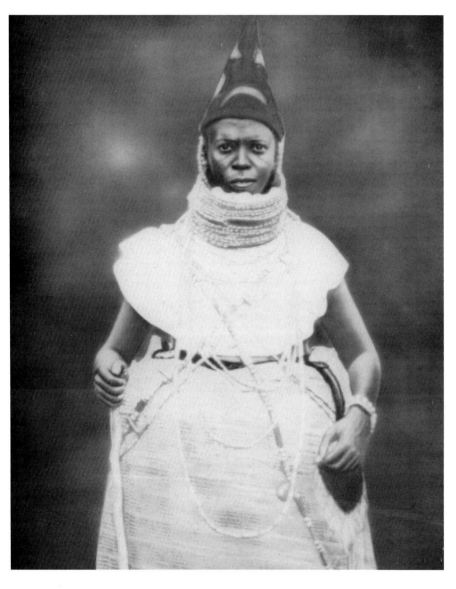

Photo of Chief Akitola, Dr. Akpata's father, in coral regalia for Ugieoba Festival.

als in various fields such as architecture, forestry, law and medicine.

Secondly, my father insisted that all his children should love and respect both family and friends. Courtesy and respect for elders was paramount since this was and still is the hallmark of Nigerian society.

My recent visit to Nigeria confirmed that this has not changed since my departure to Canada. For example, it is unacceptable for anyone to call an elder person by their first name without a prefix such as uncle or aunt, brother or sister. It is also customary to kneel or genuflect to any elder person as a sign of respect.

When we were all young, my father would summon the entire family with the ringing of a bell to meet in his quarters every morning for prayers at seven o'clock. We were not allowed under any circumstance to miss the morning prayer meeting.

It was not unusual for him to insist that we commit to memory one or two psalms to be learned within a period of one month.

My father was not only concerned about our education, our respect for our elders, obedience to the law and our faith in God, but he was also concerned about our appearance. We were all taught to shower well each morning with soap, water and a face cloth.

Our school uniforms had to be clean and well ironed before we left for school each day. He would take all of us to his tailor during special holiday occasions to be measured for a new outfit of traditional clothes. He would also take us to a shoemaker who would measure our feet to be able to make us a new pair of shoes.

These outfits were used for church, family gatherings, Easter and Christmas. In spite of the fact that this cost him a lot of money, he wanted us to look good but also loved to see the excitement on our faces when we were presented with a new outfit.

I remember Christmas as being a huge feast. My father would have two cows slaughtered for the event and the meat would first be divided between each of his sibling's families according to seniority before cooking the remainder for the family dinner.

Also, each year for my father's birthday we again had a large party of invited guests and family members. At this event, my brothers and I would be dressed in a suit and bow tie to help serve the guests. We were proud to be part of the festivities in this capacity.

Our home was quite large and built around a central courtyard. My father had separate quarters and a waiting room where he conducted business meetings. Each of us had our own bedroom.

Every day at 4 pm was tea time. My uncles and aunt as well as other friends would often come for tea and papaya or 'paw-paw' as we called it. I remember one day when my father did not want to be disturbed with other business and told me to tell any of

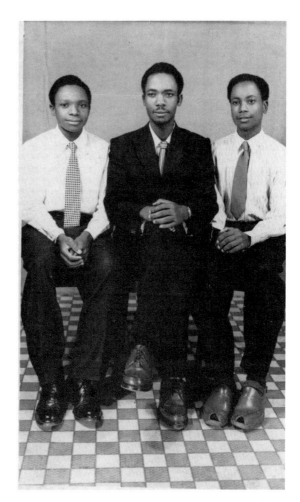

[from left] Michael, Bimbola (Frank) and Sam — brothers.

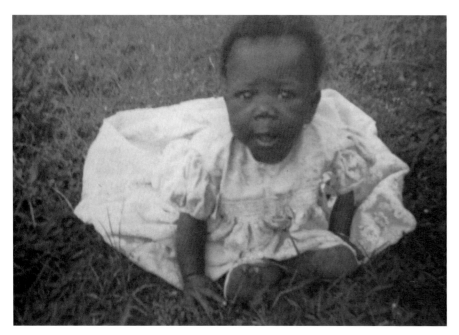

Michael as a baby in Benin City.

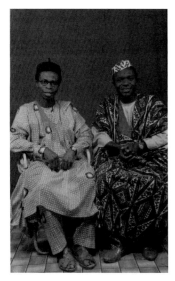

Michael [right], with a friend, in native Agbada dress.

his friends who showed up that he was not home.

Who should appear but one of my uncles who was next to my father in age. I made the terrible mistake of saying, "My father does not want to see you today." Unknown to me, he had just spoken to my dad and knew he was there. My actions resulted in six lashes to my hands from my uncle for 'misbehaving' and telling lies.

As a youngster, my best friend and playmate was my younger brother Sam. We loved to run around the house laughing and chasing each other. One day I thought I would trick him and quickly changed direction. We ran face to face into each other and he still has the scar on his cheek from my tooth hitting his face.

He is now a Professor of Dentistry and has written two books on the subject of operative dentistry. He also was the one who stayed back with our uncle and learned how to play the piano and organ.

When I was only about eight years old, my father sent me on a very unusual errand regarding his export company. One day, a shipment of my father's timber logs was loaded at the port of Sapele, a place about 30 miles from the city of Benin.

He needed the certified papers delivered to his bank in Lagos as soon as possible indicating that these logs were 'free on board' (already loaded on the ship). He placed the papers in a small bag with a strap and used two padlocks to secure it to my left wrist. We drove to the Benin airport where I boarded a DC-3 propeller plane for an hour flight to Lagos. I was told that his friend, the bank manager, would meet me at the Lagos airport to collect the package.

When I arrived, the bank manager was waiting for me and immediately took me by car to his office where he had the duplicate keys to remove the purse locked onto my left wrist. He then went to work on the papers for some time before he placed them in the same bag and locked it on my left wrist. We returned to the airport where I boarded the flight back to Benin.

My father was waiting for me at the Benin airport and quickly drove me home. There, he opened the padlocks to the small purse on my wrist and took out the papers to retrieve his payment for the logs that had been sent overseas.

These events took about four hours from the time I left Benin City and returned home. He was pleased with what I had done especially at such a young age and remarked, "You are a good son and you will go a long way in life. Thank you and may God bless you."

I was thrilled and bursting with pride because I had accomplished this mission without incident.

After a very successful and rewarding life, my father died at the age of 84. At his funeral service at the U.N.A. church cathedral in Benin City, his casket was carried into the church by representatives of the 'old boys' of King's College. During the procession into the church, these men sang the King's College school song which was quite a moving experience.

The first reading during the service was carried out by my eldest brother and the second reading was assigned to me. The text of my reading was supposed to be John 14: verses 1-10 which was a well known scripture to me. Due to my emotional upset, I read chapter 15 which was on the opposite page.

The bible was a big one and I did not realize my mistake until I was returning to my place among my family members. I felt very foolish but no one was aware of my mistake except the priest who very graciously did not say anything about it to me or anyone

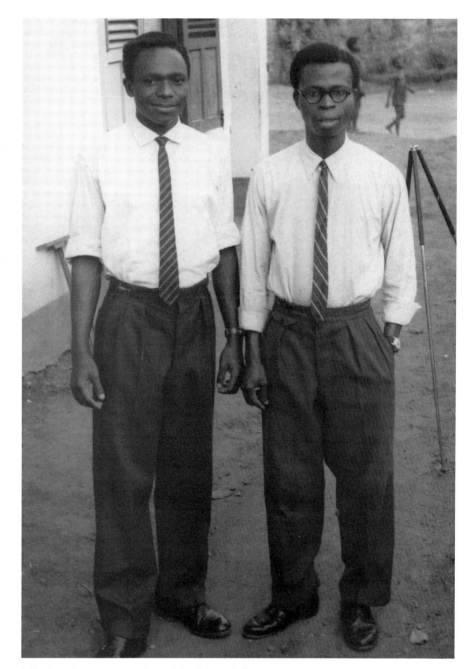

Michael at age 16, with friend Sunny Esere.

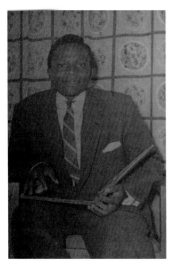

Michael, 16, his last year in Nigeria.

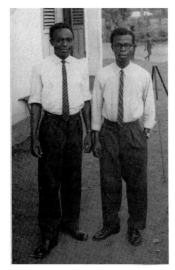

Michael [left], with a friend, in front of family home in Benin City.

else. Following the funeral service, most of the members of the church followed my family in a procession for the burial service on my father's property.

CHAPTER FORTY ONE
PRIMARY SCHOOL EDUCATION

When I was four or five years old, I started primary school. I was enrolled in Class One in a school which belonged to Uncle John Francis Akpata. 'Uncle J. F.' was next in line below my father in seniority. At the Akpata Memorial School, as it was called, I did not receive favoritism or special treatment so I worked very hard from the beginning, not to let down the family name. In all grades, I was in the top five students in the class and my uncle was very proud of me.

After four years at the Akpata Memorial School, I transferred to Eweka Memorial School owned by Uncle E. Fabiyi Akpata. 'Uncle E.F.' was my eldest uncle. This was the uncle who was the organist and pianist and the one I continued to dodge when he was trying to teach my brother and I how to play music.

While I was still attending Akpata Memorial School, I had a close call with a poisonous snake. On one hot afternoon after school was closed, I was sitting below a big mango tree waiting for my dad's driver to pick me up and take me home. I decided to pull out my arithmetic assignment and read it in preparation for completing it when I got home.

Suddenly, I heard a 'thud' beside me. I thought nothing of it as I assumed it was a mango fruit which must have dropped from the tree. But as I reached for my school bag to put my book away, my hand touched something cold that wasn't a mango fruit. I moved my hand around and finally had the nerve to look at what I was touching.

I was horrified to see a large snake curled up beside me. It did not make a move to attack me but just the sight of it filled me with terror.

I immediately jumped up and ran as fast as I could away from it, leaving my books and school bag behind. I ran home without stopping, possibly for a distance of five kilometers.

When I arrived, I ran through the door and down the hallway into my room. I slammed the door shut and fell onto the bed trembling and screaming incoherently. Everyone at home, including my father, could not understand why I did not wait at school for the driver to pick me up and was startled and afraid because of my screaming and anxiety.

Some members of the family thought that I had been attacked by a schoolmate or otherwise. I finally calmed down and at their insistence, related my story of the snake.

Everyone was surprised at what had happened and thanked God with prayers that

I had escaped an attack by a snake which they felt could have been poisonous. It must have been cold and looking for warmth next to me.

This was quite an experience which I have not forgotten. Since then, I have developed a phobia for snakes whether harmful or not. In spite of being invited to Pelee Island several times by friends, I refused to go.

I understand that snakes are very common there especially swimming in the lake. Even though they are not harmful to humans I have no desire to be near them nor am I interested in watching any snake-related movies.

Another incident that occurred during my primary school days needs to be mentioned because it was so unusual. It involved one of my school teachers at the Eweka Memorial School.

For privacy reasons, I prefer to call the teacher John. What happened between the teacher and I can best be described as bizarre.

John was my mathematics teacher and he had a younger brother in the same class with me. This younger brother was very bright. John always said that his brother had talents and abilities, which I had no reason to dispute. However, I thought it was rather unusual for a teacher to continue to sing the praises of his junior brother in the same school where he was teaching. Nevertheless, this junior brother was always one of the top students in our class.

The incident I am referring to occurred at a particular year-end examination, the results of which were to be posted on the school main notice board. Prior to the posting of the results, John was again aggrandizing his brother's prowess.

Before school was dismissed for the holidays, the results were posted. To our surprise, John's brother did not have top marks. I actually beat him by five marks, and lead the class with this result. Another young, bright boy came in second.

Needless to say, John became furious and just before I left the school, he sent a student to tell me to come to see him in his office immediately. When I got into his office, he was extremely angry and accused me of cheating in arithmetic because he thought this was the only way I could have beaten his brother by five marks. I asked him how he came to that conclusion, since he had set the examination and knew that we were both usually at the top of the class. He had no explanation.

Then he said, "I have to punish you for this offence."

He gave me six lashes with a cane. By this time the school was almost empty except for his younger brother. He said nothing about John's action.

Following the assault, as one would expect, I cried. I told John that I would report him to my uncle who was the proprietor of the school and also to a cousin of mine who was the school principal.

John became apologetic because he knew that if I carried out my threat, he would be fired from his job as a school teacher and would most likely be charged with a criminal offense.

His junior brother then approached me and apologized for his brother's actions and begged me to forgive him. I hesitated for a moment in the office and then left the room to go home and think about the entire event.

Later on, after a lot of thought, I decided not to tell my uncle or cousin about what had occurred. I was only nine years old and I have never forgotten this hateful incident. Later, word came to me that John transferred to another primary school to continue his teaching career.

CHAPTER FORTY TWO
RELATIONSHIP WITH PATIENTS AND STAFF

I was dedicated to my patients and treated each with respect and dignity. I took time during each consultation to listen carefully to what the patient had to say, and welcomed family members to be present, especially wives, as in my opinion, men are not as forthcoming with information. I especially enjoyed the challenge of solving the more difficult problems.

A sizable number of my patients were old and infirm with multiple comorbidities to the extent that I was one of the few surgeons who would want to have them as patients. I soon gained the reputation of accepting them all in my practice. Over the years I have received many letters of thanks and numerous gifts from my patients and their families which pleased my heart more than financial reward.

It also became a mystery both to my office and the hospital staff as to how I was able to calm down some of the most difficult and agitated patients and to be able to treat them with equanimity. They all saw this aspect of my practice as unique.

My relationship with hospital staff was a very humbling experience for me. Practically every hospital employee who I came in contact with during my work developed a cordial and friendly relationship with me.

No doubt, the reason this occurred was because I treated everyone with respect and showed my appreciation for their work whether they were floor cleaners, nurses, physiotherapists, clerical or administrative staff members.

It was not unusual to be stopped in the hallway on my way to the doctors' change room and met by several workers who wanted to discuss personal situations. They were always friendly and jovial but also respectful of my position as a surgeon of many years duration in the hospital.

I never showed frustration or displayed anger in any situation. I was always aware of the fact that nurses, especially those in the operating room, did their very best to make the day run effectively.

If there was ever a time that I felt I needed to speak up about a situation, I would do it in private rather than make a scene in front of others. I have always felt that we are all professional people and should be treated accordingly.

Overall, I am grateful to everyone who has helped to make my surgical practice a success, especially my office staff. I cannot say enough about the very dedicated, efficient and hard working people who have been the wheels in motion behind the scenes in the running of my office.

My secretary, Carol Attenborough, has been an invaluable asset in terms of her friendly front line contact with patients and her organizational skills in keeping everything on track in the office including myself.

I have received many letters over the years. I have chosen to include two of them.

CHAPTER FORTY THREE
REMINISCING OVER MY PRACTICE

My relationship with staff members was sincere and many have developed into close friendships. As I think back over the years, there are many stories and unusual situations to remember.

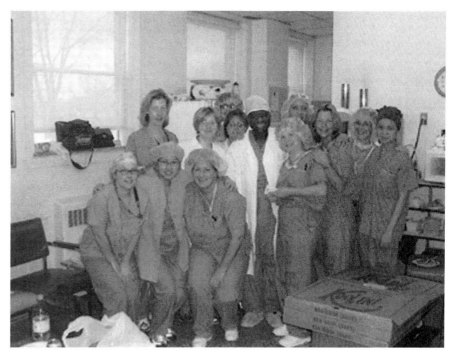

Dr. Michael Akpata with some of the operating room staff at Hôtel-Dieu Grace Hospital, 2003.

The operating room nurses at both hospitals where I did most of my work would tease me about my 'Akpatectomy' cases.

This was defined as Dr. Akpata taking on cases where the patient is critically ill with minimal chance of survival. Most often this would occur during the night requiring staff to be called in for duty. The seriousness of the situation was always discussed with the family first to involve them in the decision making process especially when the chances of success were slim.

The nurses would actually accuse me of putting out a sign directing these patients to the emergency room whenever I was on call.

Nov. 5, 2011

Dear Virginia, Dr. Akpata,

It sure was a wonderful treat to enjoy a meal together.

You both are an amazing couple kind, compassionate and caring.

Dr Akpata I have been blessed to have known you for a long time. I have the highest respect for you, not only for the great Doctor that you are but for how you interact with great compassion with everyone regardless their status.

You are a great person, anyone who is to know you will benefit by your charming and mostly warm personality. (Let us not forget, your contagious and welcoming smile).

God Bless You

Sincerely

Elena Sorrentino

Letter from Elena Sorrentino, CSR technician.

October 15, 2001

To whom it may concern.

I have had the privilege of knowing Dr. Michael Akpata for a period of 18 years at Hotel Dieu grace Hospital. As a staff nurse in the operating room and as nursing supervisor we worked together directly, often in the most critical demanding situations.

In the capacity of nursing administration, it was my responsibility to assure quality care for clients and family. Toward that end I found in Dr. Akpata a true patient advocate.

This surgeon has been consistently willing to take on the most undesirable cases, particularly the disadvantaged, vulnerable and most compromised. This significant variable is often not captured in documentation. This population is associated with the poorest outcome.

Clearly positive results are associated with good pre – op risk. Dr. Akpata assumes responsibility for the most needy surgical referrals regardless of chronic illness, social status, obesity, addiction, ability to pay, and non compliance - fully aware of *probable complication*. Other surgeons may not have.

Over the years I have known him to be consistently dedicated, knowledgeable, precise, and devoted to his work. He is also well known among the nurses for his approachable empathetic manner.

The nursing staff in the operating room and on medical surgical units, work closely with the surgeons. We are in a position to know, and have no agenda beyond patient care.

As a nursing leader I believe the veteran R.N. staff that know him best, respect Dr. Akpata and choose him for *their* families.

Sincerely,

Barbara Fitzpatrick
R.N. BSc.N. Nurse Practitioner

Letter from nurse practitioner, Barbara Fitzpatrick.

I once had a rather unkempt gentleman in his early 50s scheduled for hernia surgery later in the afternoon. He was brought down to the patient waiting area with intravenous saline running as he was in a dehydrated and emaciated state.

When the nurses went out to transport him into the operating room, they found the bed empty. Their first thought was that someone had helped him into the washroom and that he would soon return.

Upon further investigation, it was discovered that a patient had been seen leaving the hospital through a back door with an intravenous fluid running. The designated smoking area at that time was near this back door so it was not unusual for a casual observer to see a patient out there dragging an intravenous pole around as he or she was having a cigarette.

Eventually the hospital security guard found the pole on the far side of hospital property with the intravenous tubing hanging in a collection of blood. The patient was nowhere to be seen. Windsor police were notified of the situation because I wanted to be sure that he was found safely and not bleeding from the intravenous site.

Later that evening, I was notified by the police that he had been found in a downtown area but he refused to return to the hospital. He was well known to them and later taken to the Downtown Mission for food and clothes. Unfortunately after this event, every effort made by my office to contact this gentleman was unsuccessful.

Another case involved a gentleman booked for surgery who took the food tray from his room partner who was sleeping when it was delivered. When the nurse entered the room to transport him to the operating room, she was shocked to see him sitting up in a chair eating, even though he had been instructed not to have anything before his surgery.

I was notified immediately and went to visit him between my cases in the operating room to find out what had happened. When asked why he took the food, he just said he was hungry and it was not fair that his roommate had received food and he did not.

He was rebooked for his surgery as the first case in the morning so the hospital staff could keep a better eye on him.

Removing foreign bodies from the esophagus, stomach and rectum is not an uncommon event but I soon gained the reputation of having some of the strangest items whenever I was on call for emergency coverage.

Most often it was a bolus of partially chewed food that was caught in the esophagus which can be dangerous especially if it obstructs the windpipe. If it is in the lower part of the esophagus it can often be pushed down into the stomach with a gastroscope.

I once had a case dealing with a man having a piece of chicken bone lodged in his

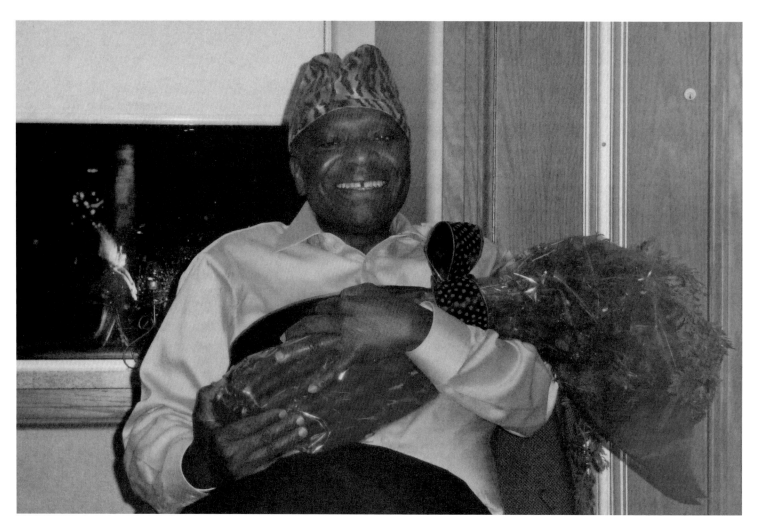

A bouquet of carrots given to Dr. Akpata as a joke by the nursing staff at his retirement party.

esophagus near the entrance to the stomach. Pushing it through was not an option because the bone could tear the esophagus, and that could require surgery.

With the careful use of forceps to turn the piece of bone, a basket retriever was passed over a guide wire to enclose and eventually remove it. I then had to reinsert the scope to check the area in order to make sure that there was no injury to the mucosa or obstruction caused by a tumor.

I have removed coins, marbles and many other items from the stomach which were accidentally swallowed, or illicit drugs hidden in condoms for illegal transport across the Canadian border to the U.S.

These drug-filled condoms are swallowed and eventually pass through the bowel to be retrieved at a later date. The danger of course is the possibility of rupture of any of them during this process. It has happened that patients have had surgery resulting in a temporary colostomy after the removal of several bags of cocaine from various levels of the bowel.

The list of other items I have removed from the bowel over the years includes such things as a small juice bottle, an old style television tube with prongs, an after shave bottle, a beer bottle and various odd shaped vegetables including a carrot.

As you can imagine, I became the 'butt' of many jokes throughout the hospital. The nurses in the operating room were relentless in the teasing with such comments as 'What's up Doc?' and 'When is the next carrotectomy?'

At my retirement party, instead of receiving flowers, I was given a bouquet of carrots and a necktie with pictures of carrots on it. The bouquet was tied nicely with a ribbon, and I had to wear the necktie for the rest of the evening. This again is an example of the comfortable relationship that I had with the majority of the staff members.

CHAPTER FORTY FOUR
PASSIONS IN LIFE

My passions in life include the following: work, family, religion, classical music and politics.

MY WORK

Anyone who knows me well cannot deny the fact that I have a passion for medicine, especially surgery. From what you have already read, it should be quite obvious that my work has been the central focus of my life.

Since entering medical school, I have dedicated myself to studying and learning in earnest in order to keep on top of any new advances to be able to provide the best care to my patients.

In Windsor, I have spent an inordinate number of hours attempting to help my patients return to normal health, often to the detriment of my family life. The patients

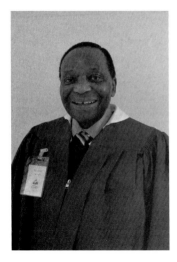

Dr. Akpata in his St. James Anglican Church choir uniform.

who were referred to me came from all walks of life, various backgrounds and different personalities.

I treated each patient with great compassion and tried not to prejudge anyone. Every step was taken to make sure that the cause of their problem was diagnosed and the proper treatment prescribed. Invariably most of my patients developed implicit confidence in me which translated into good treatment results and often led to long standing friendships.

MY FAMILY

The deep love I have for my family is unending. My eldest son Michael was born just as I was beginning my residency training program in general surgery at the University of Alberta. These were some difficult years in terms of the time I was available to spend with my family as I was on call for long stretches. Michelle was born two years after that and John followed approximately two years later.

They were all subject to the rigors of the dedication I had to my work.

During their formative years, I participated as much as possible in their care but most of their upbringing was done by their mother. In spite of my love for my family, the demand and intensity of my practice led to what I prefer to call 'benign neglect'. I spent less time with my family, which is the biggest regret regarding my surgical practice.

During my retirement party, my eldest son, Michael, had the opportunity to give a speech about me. He alluded to the fact that he remembered the many occasions when our family was ready to sit down at the dinner table to eat when I was called out to attend to a sick patient. Often this occurred during our Christmas dinner.

I hope and pray that my children have forgiven me for my limited presence in their daily affairs as they were growing up. I am indeed grateful to God that my children are very bright and well-educated. They have grown up to be adults who are respected among their peers and in their respective communities as a whole.

MY RELIGION

I was born into a Christian family, baptized and then confirmed in the Anglican Church. My grandfather and my eldest uncles were pianists and organists in our church in Benin City. At the early age of six, my brother and I were already in the church choir.

When I arrived in Canada, I continued to attend the Anglican Church throughout my university days. As time passed, my work became a priority and I attended church services less regularly.

At one point, a close medical colleague who noticed the tension in my life encour-

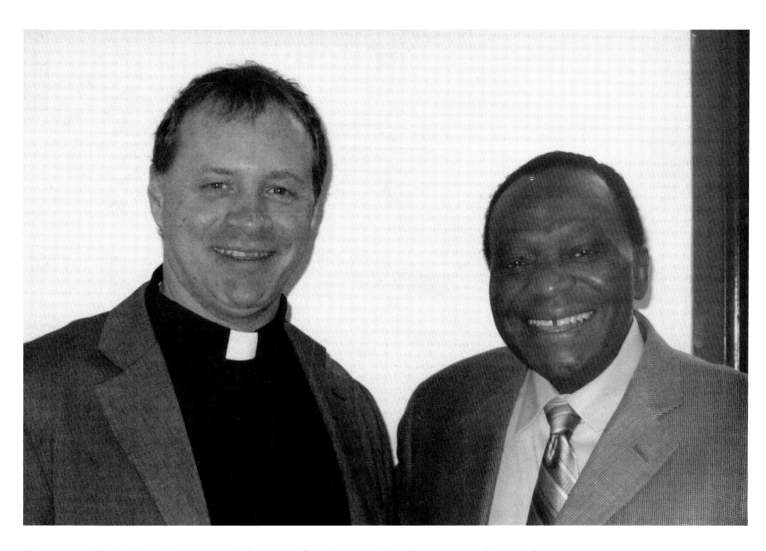

Reverend Rob Henderson, minister of St. James Anglican church and Dr. Michael Akpata.

aged me to attend his church as he felt that I needed to focus my attention more on the spiritual aspect of my life. I am grateful to him for noticing and helping me to regroup myself.

Eventually, I returned to my own denomination as an Anglican, and today I continue to read my Bible daily as I had done in the past. Since retirement, I have become much more involved in church activities. I also resumed memorizing certain passages of the Bible which have helped me deal with situations arising in my life.

Some of these are as follows:

- Psalm 37: verses 23-25 "The steps of a good man are ordered by the Lord; and he delighteth in his way. Though he may fall, he shall not be utterly cast down; for the Lord upholdeth him with his hand. I have been young and now am old; yet have I not seen the righteous forsaken, nor his seed begging bread."

- Isaiah 41: verse 31 "But they that wait upon the Lord shall renew their strength; they shall mount up with wings as eagles; they shall run, and not be weary; and they shall walk, and not faint."

- Deuteronomy 31: verse 6 "Be strong and of a good courage, fear not, nor be afraid of them; for the Lord thy God, he it is that doth go with thee; he will not fail thee, nor forsake thee."

- Sirach 2: verses 4-6 "Accept whatever happens to you. Even if you suffer humiliation, be patient. Gold is tested by fire, and human character is tested in the furnace of humiliation. Trust the Lord, and he will help you. Walk straight in his ways, and put your hope in him."

CLASSICAL MUSIC

Unfortunately when I was six years old, I preferred to run away and play soccer instead of learning the organ and piano from my eldest uncle. I now regret this lost opportunity. Luckily for my brother, he latched on to my uncle's call and now he plays for his church on a regular basis.

As I have grown older, I have come to realize that my interest and aptitude for classical music is almost equal to my love of medicine. This remark is not an exaggeration and I envy the concert pianists for their talents.

When I was at King's College, we were taught classical music appreciation which was held once a week for one hour. During this session, each student in the class would be asked by our teacher to follow in our mind a particular instrument in the music being played. At the end of the music program, we were questioned individually as to the role of that specific instrument in the piece. No talking or fidgeting in the class was allowed during the recital.

In addition, we were taught the history of classical music, and the life histories of each of the composers. This class, combined with my family background in music led to the development of my intense interest in this type of music.

I prefer classical to any other type of music as it helps me relax, work better with people, control anxiety and fall asleep with ease. In fact, I usually listen to a piano or violin sonata for about an hour before going to bed at night. My favorite choices are those by Beethoven, Mozart and Franz Schubert, although it is hard to find a piece of music or composer prior to the twentieth century that I do not like.

This may sound very odd, coming from someone who was born in Nigeria where traditional and ethnic music was endemic. However my passion is unquestionable.

POLITICS

The word politics comes from the Greek word, Politikos, meaning, 'of, for or relating to citizens'. More specifically, it refers to the organized control of a community of people whether within a city, state or country. Over time, there have been many different political systems around the world including parliamentary or presidential democracy, communism, despotism, totalitarianism or autocratic government.

In all these instances, only democracy has the interest of the people at heart and this is supported by the constitution of the involved countries. By definition, democracy is 'the government of the people, for the people and by the people'. Therefore the government has to take into account the wishes of the entire country's population, regardless of their political leanings.

In Canada, we have the freedom, safety, and all the necessary amenities to live a good life. We do not have to be worried about unnecessary harassment by the government.

In my opinion, this is the main difference between democracy and many other forms of government. I dare say however, that for this very reason most Canadians do not participate in politics the way they should because they are very comfortable and feel secure.

As a result of this apathy, it behooves journalists to become the caretakers of society by bringing public opinions on specific matters to the attention of the leaders as to their role in the government.

In this day and age of mass communication, it is also necessary for the average person in the country to express his or her opinion in a free and unrestrictive way on matters of great importance to the society.

CONCLUSION

I have had a great and satisfying life both as a youngster in Nigeria where I was born and in Canada where I have lived most of my life. I have had God's blessings in every aspect of my life. I feel that I have contributed a great deal to the field of medicine particularly in Windsor and have served my patients well, many of whom have become my friends.

In Canada, I have lived a safe and secure life, better than in many other countries in the world, even though there were moments when I felt I would have been financially better off elsewhere.

My profession was not designed for financial reward but rather to look after the sick. The talents we have as doctors or surgeons should not prioritize money over helping to save lives.

I have enjoyed most of my time in Windsor but looking back, the time I spent at the University of Alberta was equally happy and exciting. I am grateful for the people I have met and the relationships that have developed over the years. That is what I miss the most about retirement. I've been blessed with three children and four grandchildren which makes it even more pleasant and fruitful for me.

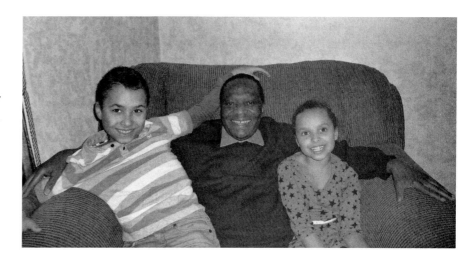

Michael Akpata with his two grandchildren Reece and Regan.

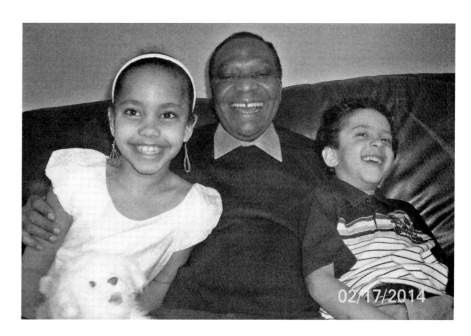

Michael Akpata with his two grandchildren Ayla and Evan.

ACKNOWLEDGEMENTS

I would like to acknowledge Virginia Whittal for her intense commitment to this book. She was able to transcribe my hand-written notes into a legible manuscript and it grew from there. Art Stone for his advice and contributions toward the writing of this book. Mike Busuttil for his computer expertise, and Bob Meyer for his dedication to editing, and ensuring that this book was well formulated in an orderly manner—the words second to none. Finally, I would like to thank Black Moss Press: Marty Gervais, Vanessa Shields and Jason Rankin for their dedication and patience as we worked through the process of publishing this book.

PRAISE FOR LIFE BEHIND THE MASK

Dr. Michael Akpata tells an inspirational story as he leads the reader through his early life and educational path, and ultimately into his professional life as a surgeon at the forefront of advancements in general surgery. Dr. Akpata was instrumental in the development of laser surgery, surgical stapling, minimally invasive surgery and advanced laparoscopic surgery in Windsor and beyond.

Life Behind the Mask: A Surgeon's Memoir is Dr. Akpata's journey, filled with insights and reflections on a professional life lived. It is the story of a man who has left a lasting legacy for surgeons who follow. A captivating read for anyone interested in the history and progress of general surgery in Windsor.

— Dr. Charles Pearce, M.D.

I have known Michael for many years. The book reflects his personality so well, particularly his sincerity. The dedication to his patients stands out in my mind. I can vouch for this because any time I went out to dinner with Michael and Virginia there was always somebody that came to the table to give him a hug and thank him for saving their life with his surgical skills. It must have been such a rewarding career. Thank God there are such dedicated persons in our medical system.

— Rev. Peter Aquilina

My memories of Dr. Akpata during my career at Hotel-Dieu Grace Hospital are of a man who was always professional, respectful of others, who genuinely took an interest in people, and who treated everyone the same. He cared deeply for his patients and in an effort to help anyone he could, he seemed to take on patients that other surgeons might not. His story, Life Behind the Mask: A Surgeon's Memoir gives insight into how his upbringing, education, experiences, beliefs and convictions, helped mould him into such a caring man and respected surgeon.

— John Coughlin, former Senior Vice-President of Hotel Dieu Hospital